**WELL**YOUR WORLD

# EAT YOUR BEST IN 10 MINUTES OR LESS

**REEBS & DILLON HOLMES**

OUR FAVORITE PLANT-BASED RECIPES | SALT, OIL, & SUGAR FREE

EAT YOUR BEST IN 10 MINUTES OR LESS

© Reebs & Dillon Holmes 2025

https://wellyourworld.com

All Rights Reserved. No part of this book may be used or reproduced in any manner whatsoever without written permission. You may print the pages of this digital book for personal use only.

Print Edition ISBN # 978-1-962540-98-8
Digital Edition ISBN # 978-1-962540-99-5

The ideas, concepts, recipes, and opinions expressed in this book are intended to be used for educational purposes only. Our books and recipes are sold with the understanding that author and publisher are not rendering medical advice of any kind, nor are the books or recipes intended to replace medical advice, nor to diagnose, prescribe or treat any disease, condition, illness, or injury.

It is imperative that before beginning any diet or exercise program, including any aspects of this book, you receive full medical clearance from a qualified physician.

Authors claim no responsibility to any person or entity for any liability, loss, or damage caused or alleged to be caused directly or indirectly as a result of the use, application, or interpretation of the material in this book.

# WELL YOUR WORLD!

It's been quite a journey for me since joining Well Your World in 2019. When I came on board, our popular live cooking show membership was in its infancy, Dillon had only been on YouTube for a couple years, and he was just getting started selling a few healthy food products. Dillon and I have learned and grown along the way, with you by our side, and we are so appreciative of your support.

One thing that challenged us in the beginning was coming up with the right recipes for our live cooking show and YouTube videos. We figured people wanted the typical "fancy" cookbook recipes, but the truth was that wasn't how we ate at home. Sure, we enjoy making an elaborate meal from scratch occasionally, but what we really ate were easy meals like Starch Blaster (YouTube Favorites Vol. 2 cookbook) or our Mexican Buddha Bowl (page 49) - a delicious Latin-inspired dish made with easy-to-find freezer and pantry staples. And to our surprise, those quick, easy recipes became our most popular! It felt like we truly found our tribe...real people who are more passionate about their health than about recipe flare or elaborate multi-course meals.

I'll be honest, when I first proposed a "10 Minute Meals" cooking show episode, Dillon thought I was crazy (which I am). He was not sure that anyone would want to make meals as simple as the ones WE eat day to day, but like any good husband, he humored me. And sure enough, the positive feedback we received from our community after our initial show was ASTOUNDING. The first five 10-Minute Meals we created (McReebs Wrap, Potato Corn Chowder, Peanut Ramen Bowl, Mexican Buddha Bowl, Chickpea Lettuce Cups) also hit viral status on our YouTube channel compared to our normal recipe videos.

That was a pivotal moment because it provided so much insight into what our community actually wanted: simple, health-promoting meals that get us in and out of the kitchen fast, made with affordable, no-fuss ingredients you can find almost anywhere.

Because the quick recipes in this book reflect the way we actually eat, I'm proud to say this is our favorite cookbook so far. We've never felt more aligned with our vibrant community. Thank you from the bottom of our hearts for supporting us, not just financially, but with all of the kind comments, requests, and feedback you've provided us over the years. Our "joie de vivre," joy of life, is hearing the positive impact that our work has had on your life and your health. We hope you enjoy the recipes in this book as much as we enjoy eating them every day.

xoxo, Reebs

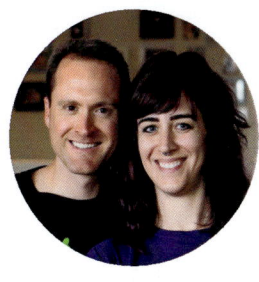

- 🌐 www.wellyourworld.com
- ▶ youtube.com/@wellyourworld
- f facebook.com/groups/wellyourworld
- 📷 @wellyourworld
- ✉ hello@wellyourworld.com

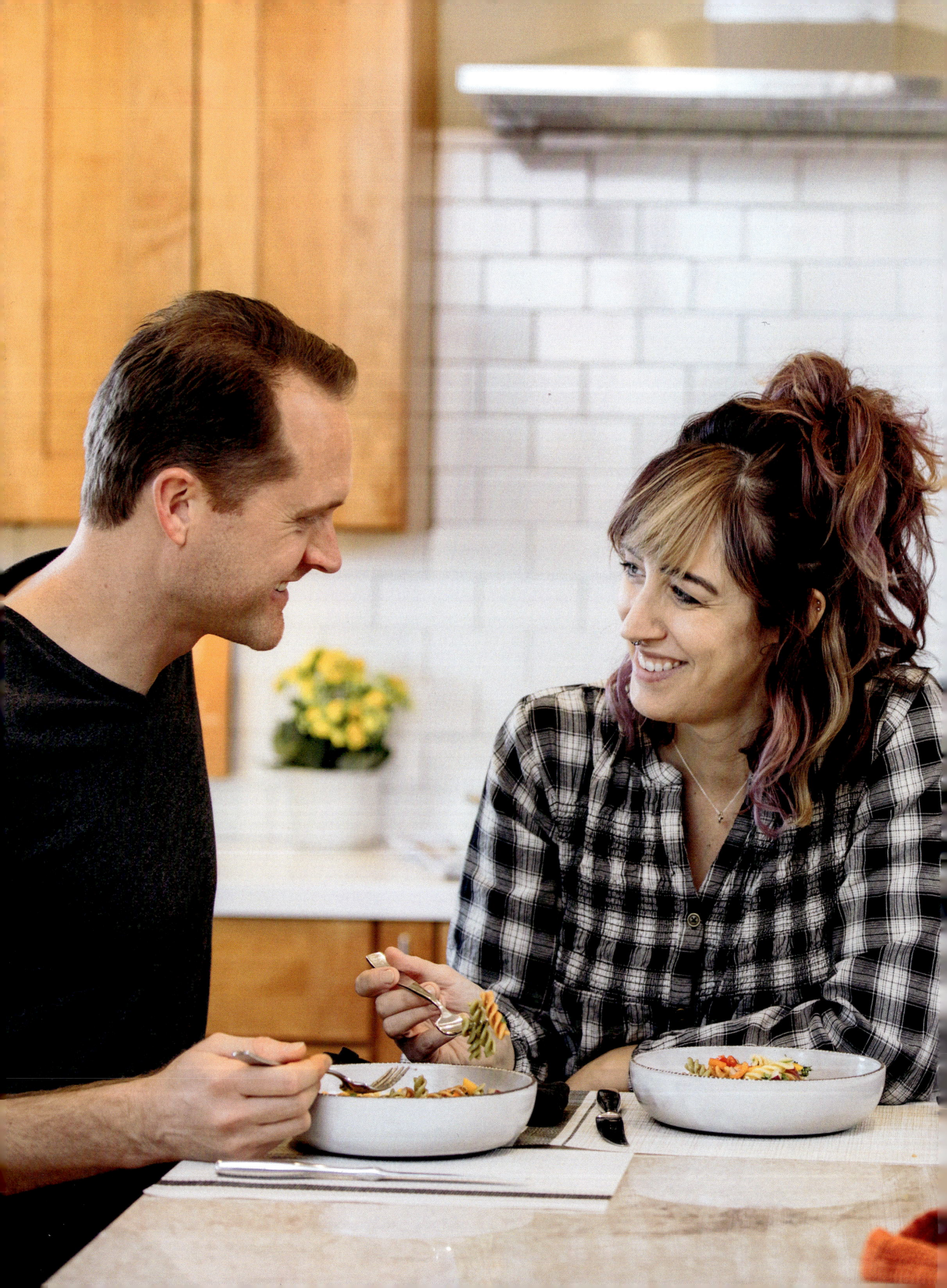

# SETTING THE RECORD STRAIGHT

## THE WORLD IS IN A HEALTH CRISIS, AND FOOD IS THE CULPRIT.

It's clear that there is a health epidemic of preventable and reversible illness. For most, it starts with high blood pressure and cholesterol and quickly leads to obesity, type 2 diabetes, and various cancers and autoimmune disorders. We can battle these diseases with each and every bite, because the food we put in our mouths makes all the difference.

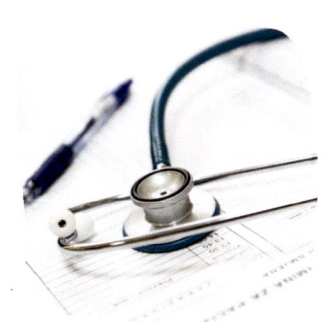

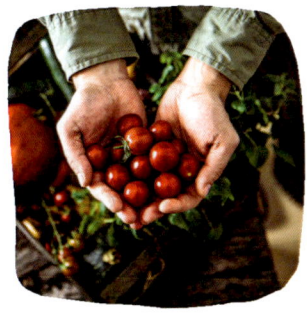

## WE DIDNT GET SICK FROM DIETARY DEFICIENCY.

Too many "experts" push a plant-based approach which requires absolute perfection. This is overwhelming and unsustainable for most people. Instead of worrying about extracting every last vitamin and mineral from our food, we are better off focusing on what we REMOVE: excessive animal products and highly processed, hyper-palatable foods.

## NO ONE HAS TIME TO SPEND ALL DAY IN THE KITCHEN.

People often believe you have to create a perfectly balanced plate at every meal, complete with super-food ingredients and complex cooking steps. The truth is that health comes from enjoying a wide variety of whole, natural foods prepared easily and quickly. Simplicity is the key to creating a sustainable lifestyle. Want to get fancy? Save it for the weekend or special occasions.

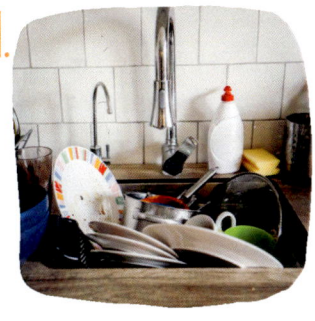

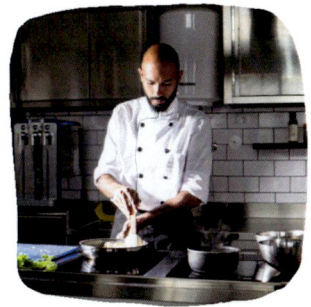

## YOU DONT HAVE TO BE A CHEF TO CREATE TASTY MEALS THAT PROMOTE YOUR HEALTH AND SAVE TIME.

Transitioning to a simple, plant-based diet is easier than most people realize. Cooking shouldn't require elaborate chef-y techniques or extensive food knowledge. Sure there might be a small learning curve if you're not used to preparing your own meals, but we eliminate the extra steps and follow a simple, standardized Well Your World approach to cooking.

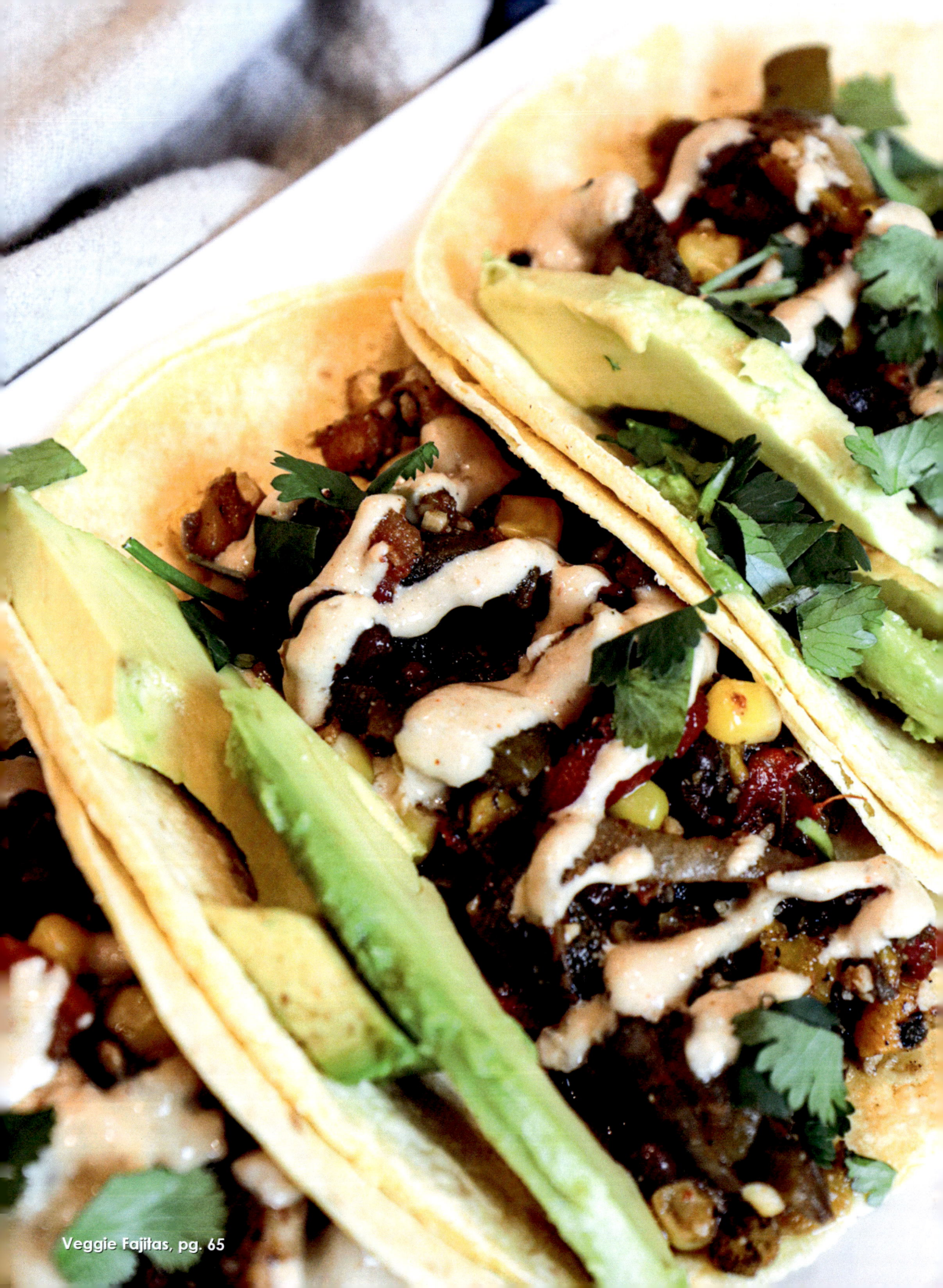
Veggie Fajitas, pg. 65

# WHAT SETS US APART

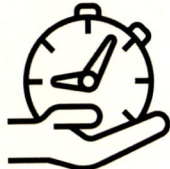 Our recipes are the fastest in the plant-based world. You won't find any other plant-based meals, free of processed junk like salt, oil, and sugar, that are faster or simpler to whip up than ours. That is also why we invented our time-saving food products, to help even the busiest people maintain a sustainable, healthy diet.

Frozen, canned, and other convenience foods (always simple, whole food ingredients) are common in our dishes. Let's be real, not everyone has time to chop or shop for fresh veggies. Things like frozen potatoes, bell peppers, and other vegetables are lifesavers for this way of eating.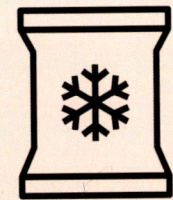

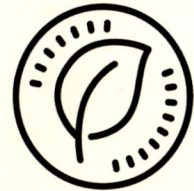 We don't stress about things like whether or not our ingredients are totally organic. It is a great thing to strive for, but not everyone has the access or funds to eat a totally organic diet. Remember, it wasn't eating non-organic vegetables that got us into the widespread health crisis we're in now; it was overconsumption of processed foods and animal products that did this to us.

We skip traditional cooking steps as much as possible in our recipes. For example, if sautéing the veggies only adds about 5% more flavor but takes 20% more time, then it's just not worth it. We keep it simple, easy, and approachable for all.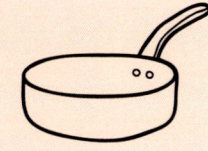

 Our recipes are loved by veterans and newbies alike. You don't have to be an expert to put together a tasty meal for you and your family. Many of our recipes are dump-and-go which anyone can do and everyone will appreciate!

Despite the corners we cut in our cooking, we don't skimp on flavor. When you reduce or eliminate sugar, oil, and salt, you need extra herbs and spices to amp up the taste, and we don't hold back! You'll find that our dishes are delicious despite how easy and simple they are to prepare. Spend time experimenting to discover the flavors you enjoy, and then just play the hits over and over.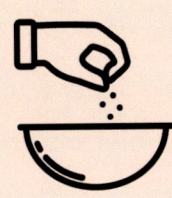

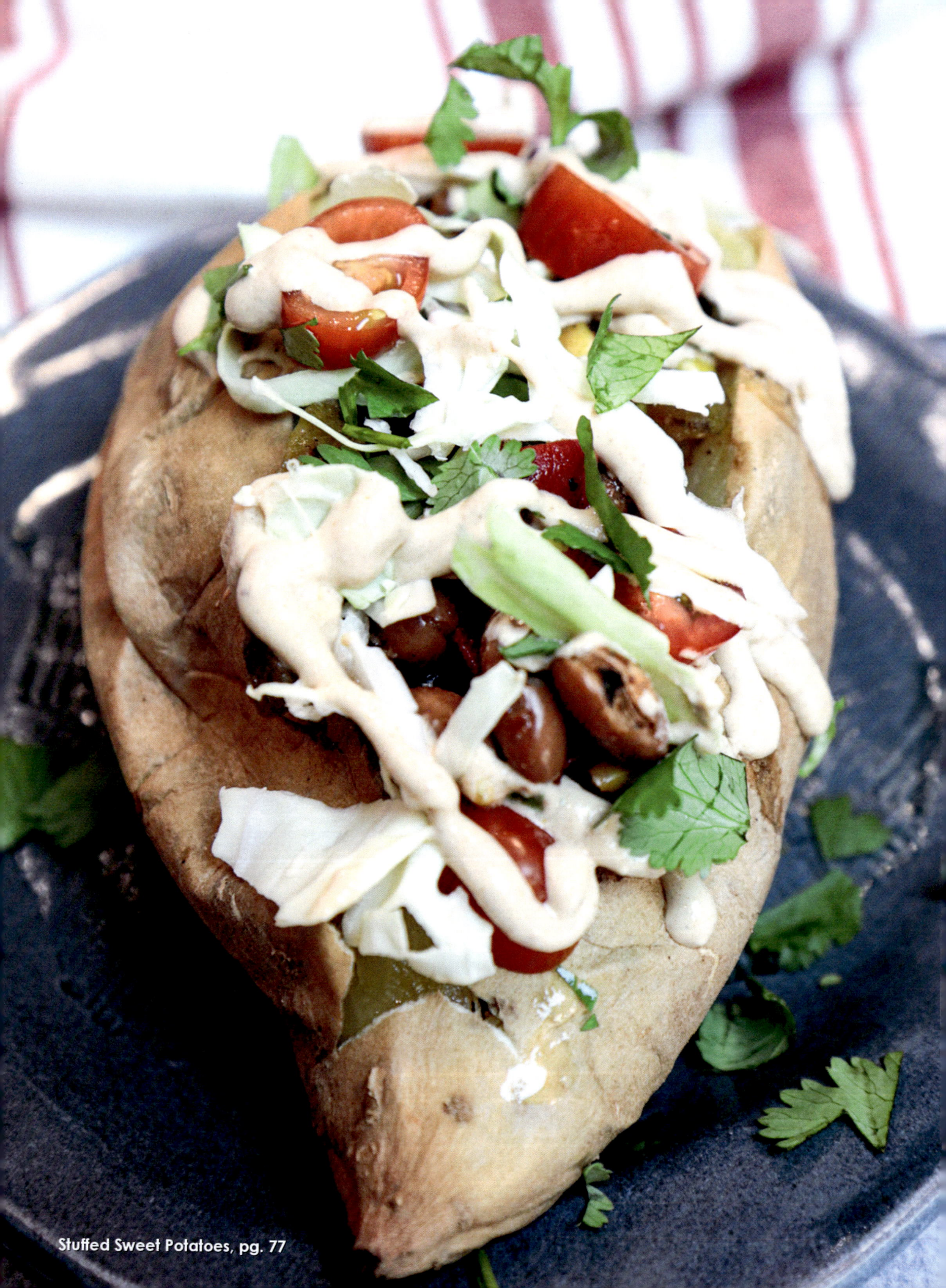
Stuffed Sweet Potatoes, pg. 77

# THE PERFECTION TRAP

## MEALS DON'T NEED MULTIPLE COURSES OR DISHES

When coming from a Standard American Diet (SAD), we are used to our plates looking a certain way. Most people believe there must be a soup course, a salad, the main dish, and even more sides. Some people think of building their plates as a protein, a vegetable, and a grain. Here, we just cook simple, health-promoting meals and eat them. You'll have plenty to eat and lots of variety, so eliminate the pressure of "tradition" and free yourself to enjoy a simple one-bowl meal!

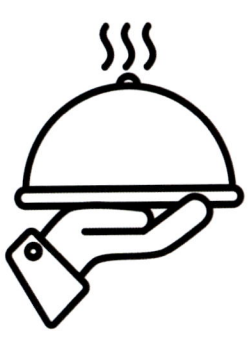

## SAVE FANCY SPREADS FOR THE WEEKENDS

You don't have to cook complex, multi-step recipes, such as lasagna, stuffed peppers, or tamales. You can enjoy easier versions of these classics like pasta with our WYW pasta sauces, our Stuffed Pepper Soup, or our Tamale Pie which deliver the same nostalgic flavors in a fraction of the time. We love to cook but we save the fancy stuff for the weekends.

## DON'T GET OVERWHELMED TRYING TO FOLLOW STRICT PLANT-BASED DOCTRINES

It can be information overload when you first decide to adopt a plant-based diet. Not all of the doctors we respect agree on every tiny detail, which can make it even more confusing. You will hear some "experts" say you MUST eat certain foods EVERY DAY to maintain optimal health. That just isn't true. Our bodies are very efficient at extracting what we need when we need it, so instead of focusing on what you eat in a day, focus on the variety of whole, natural foods you enjoy all week.

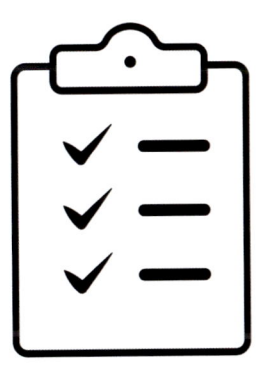

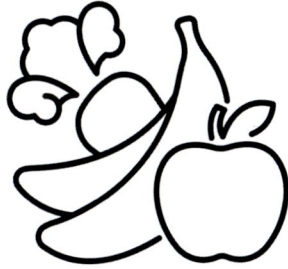

## FOCUS ON THE BIG PICTURE, NOT THE TINY DETAILS

People tend to focus too much on small, minute details instead of the big picture. These distractions often pull us away from our routine and make adhering to our way of eating more stressful and intimidating than necessary. If we shift our focus to ensuring we eat a variety of simple, healthy meals based on starches, vegetables, and fruit, we can achieve great health without worrying about the pressure of perfection.

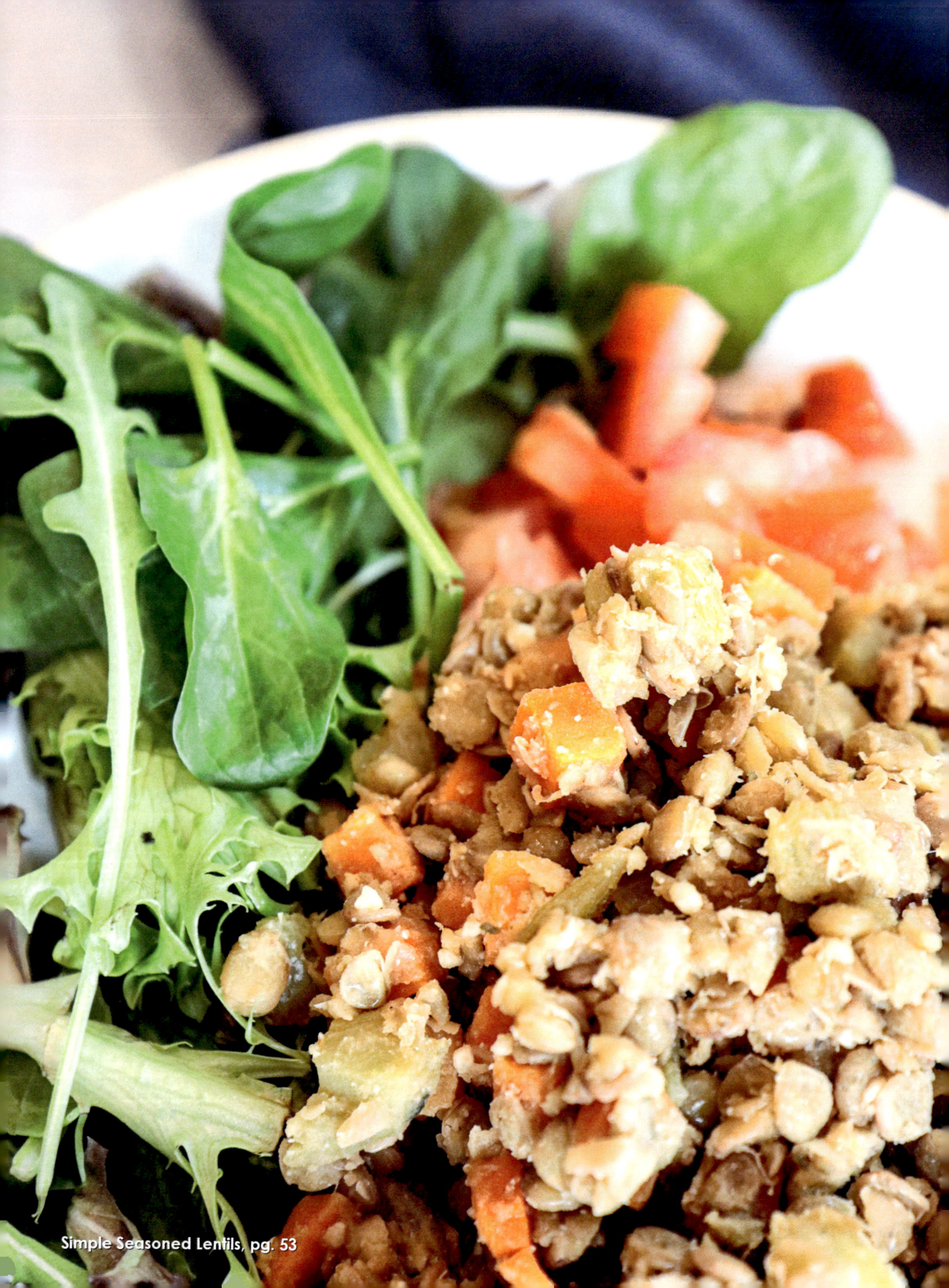
Simple Seasoned Lentils, pg. 53

# WHAT IS "RECIPE AMNESIA" AND HOW TO BEAT IT!

You've probably never heard the term "recipe amnesia" before, and that's because Reebs invented it! But I AM sure you've experienced it over and over again. It's that feeling when you've spent a hard day working, either at the office, or at home, taking care of your kids or grandchildren, and then mealtime rolls around and you suddenly forget every healthy meal you've ever made. The fridge and pantry are full, but you have no idea what to eat. Have you been there? We have, which is embarrassing because we've cooked over 700 recipes on our live cooking show and on YouTube!

Some people may think we're referring to "decision fatigue" which is another buzz phrase these days, and yes they are related! But recipe amnesia is what comes AFTER decision fatigue. Let me explain...

A typical day for us consists of getting the kids ready in the morning, driving them to school, getting to work answering emails, working on projects, and so on. SO MUCH mental energy is spent making important decisions, and by the time it comes down to picking which meal to make, we don't have any more brain energy left! This is why food simplicity is so important.

To stick to this way of eating you need to make it completely brainless. That's why we encourage you to have a place where you can view your current favorite EASY recipes, such as on your fridge or inside your pantry door. We call this your meal rotation, and it should only consist of about half a dozen meals at a time. Gone are the days of complicated meal planners and loads of recipes to choose from. Here is the solution...

## HOW TO BEAT RECIPE AMNESIA:

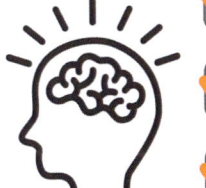

 **Figure out your shopping list basics and always have those on hand.**

 **Have an area where you can view your favorite recipes at a glance.**

 **Cut out the recipe cards in the back of this book and choose 6-8.**

 **Stick those recipes to your fridge to make your meal rotation.**

 **Recipe amnesia? Simply pick from your new rotation and enjoy!**

 **Play the hits! Don't be afraid to enjoy the same meals on repeat.**

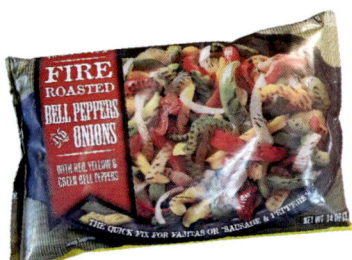 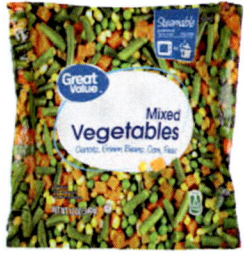 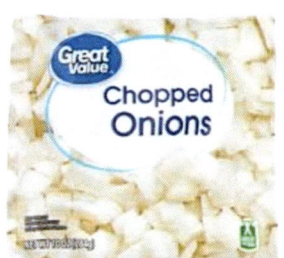 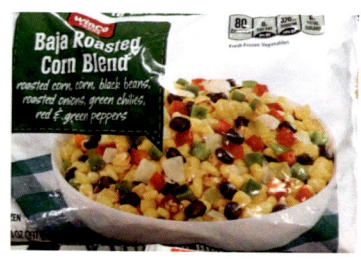
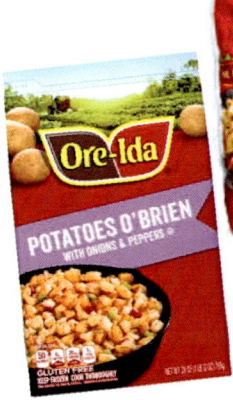 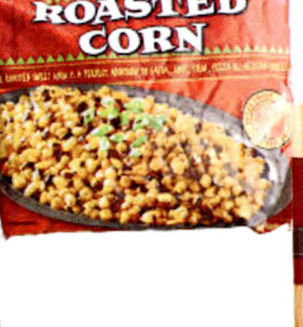 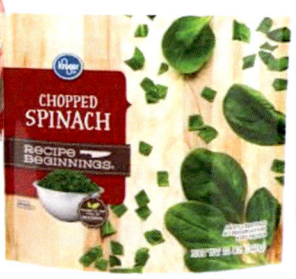 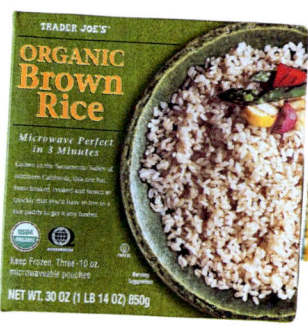 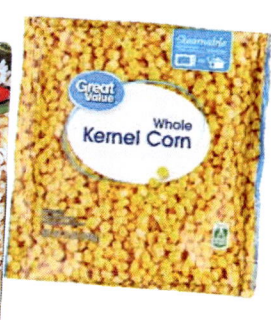

# OUR FAVORITE PANTRY & FREEZER PRODUCTS

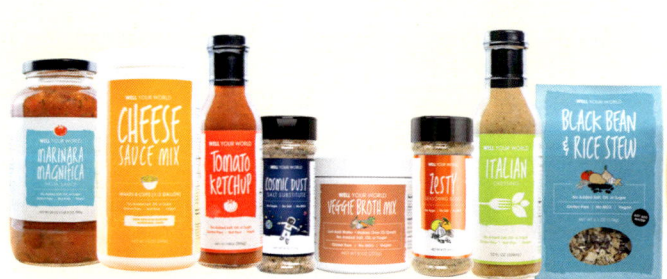

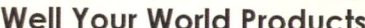

Well Your World Products

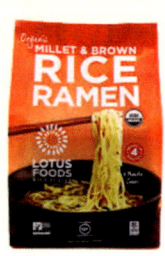 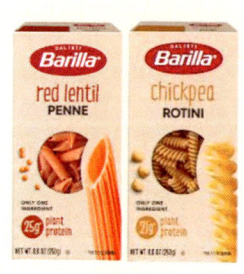

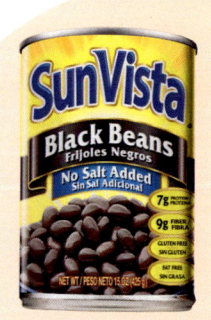 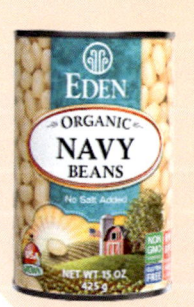 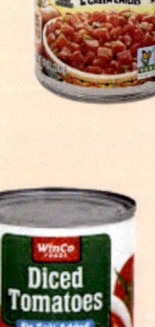 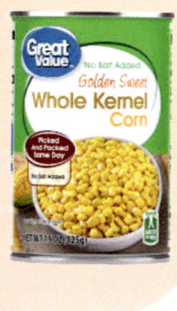

# SOME "10 MINUTE" COOKING HACKS

We pride ourselves on using cooking shortcuts that save time without sacrificing flavor. Here are some of the most common hacks we perform in the kitchen.

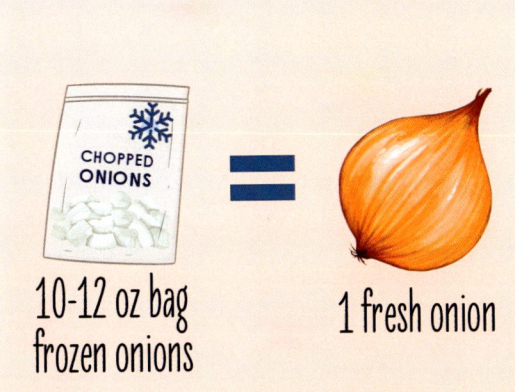

10-12 oz bag frozen onions = 1 fresh onion

A good rule of thumb for single ingredient frozen vegetables is that you can usually count on one frozen bag being about equal to one of the chopped fresh version. With this information, you can easily swap these items either direction in your own cooking.

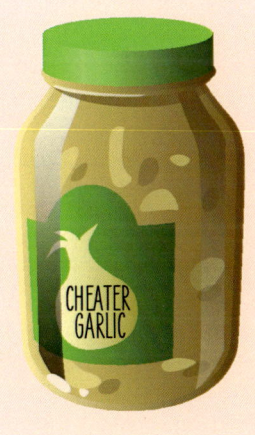

We aren't afraid to use things like cheater garlic around here. Cheater garlic is the jarred minced garlic usually found in the produce section. It's not as potent as fresh garlic, but it sure does save time. Just use a little extra!

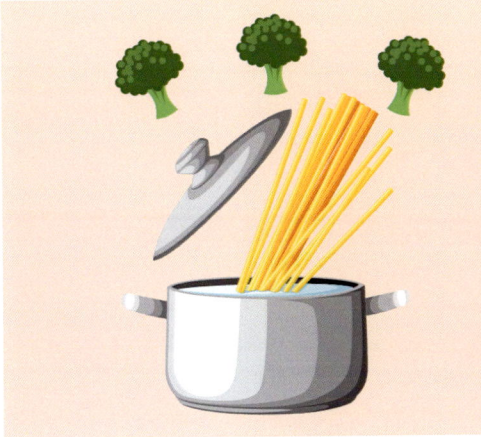

Another hack we absolutely love is adding fresh or frozen vegetables to our pasta cooking water for the last couple minutes of simmering. It's such a fast, easy way to add more veggies to things like pasta & sauce or our mac & cheese using our world famous WYW Cheese Sauce Mix.

# WHAT DOES IT MEAN TO EAT HEALTHY?

We promote a diet based on whole, natural foods, free of animal products including meat, fish, fowl, eggs, and dairy products. We also dramatically reduce our salt, oil, and sugar intake. Why? Because this way of eating allows you to get back to your body's natural weight and maintain great health, all while feeling full and satisfied at every meal. Say goodbye to calorie counting and portion control.

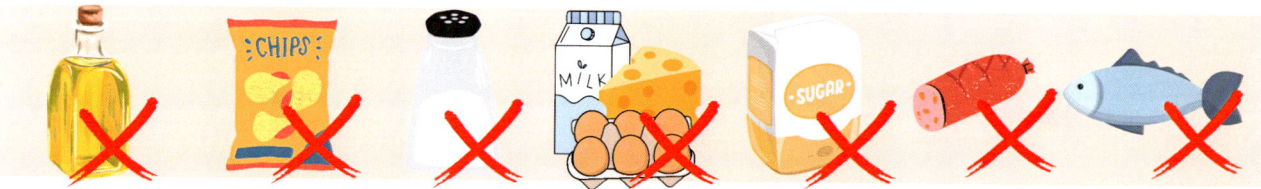

You can see from the WYW Food Pyramid below that we get the bulk of our calories from whole, satiating starches like potatoes, rice, beans, and lentils...our body's natural, primary fuel source. Non-starchy veggies and fresh fruit provide flavor, nutrient density, and variety. We top off with a small amount of whole natural fats like nuts, seeds, avocado, and soy (tofu, edamame). We also enjoy small amounts of lightly processed foods like whole grain bread or dried fruit.

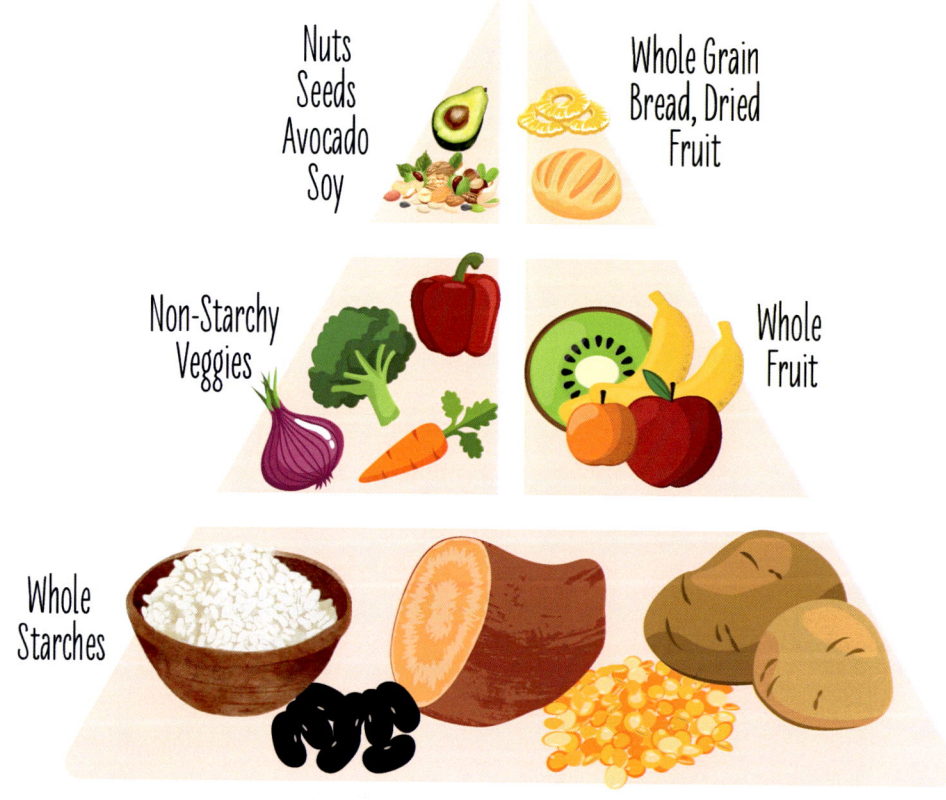

# THE CALORIE DENSITY CHART

Calorie density defines how CONCENTRATED a food is. It is usually measured as calories per pound. But you could also think of it as calories per mouthful or even calories per meal. Understanding the relative difference between the various foods is more important than the unit of measure.

The point of understanding calorie density is to help you consume large amounts of food without consuming too many calories. You don't want to feel hungry all the time by consuming too little volume or by trying to eat rich foods "in moderation."

To utilize calorie density to your advantage, eliminate the ultra-rich foods such as oils, processed junk foods, and animal products. Instead, eat freely on a diet of leafy greens, veggies, fresh fruit, and whole starches like grains, legumes, and tubers. Be careful not to overdo it on the healthy fats like nuts/seeds/avocado/soy in order to maintain your body's natural weight. Those rich foods should just be used to add flavor, so don't make them the centerpiece of your meal.

One way of using this calorie density "hack" is to begin each meal with a salad or soup to fill up on foods that are more calorie dilute before moving on to more calorie dense staples like cooked starches with some whole fats for flavor.

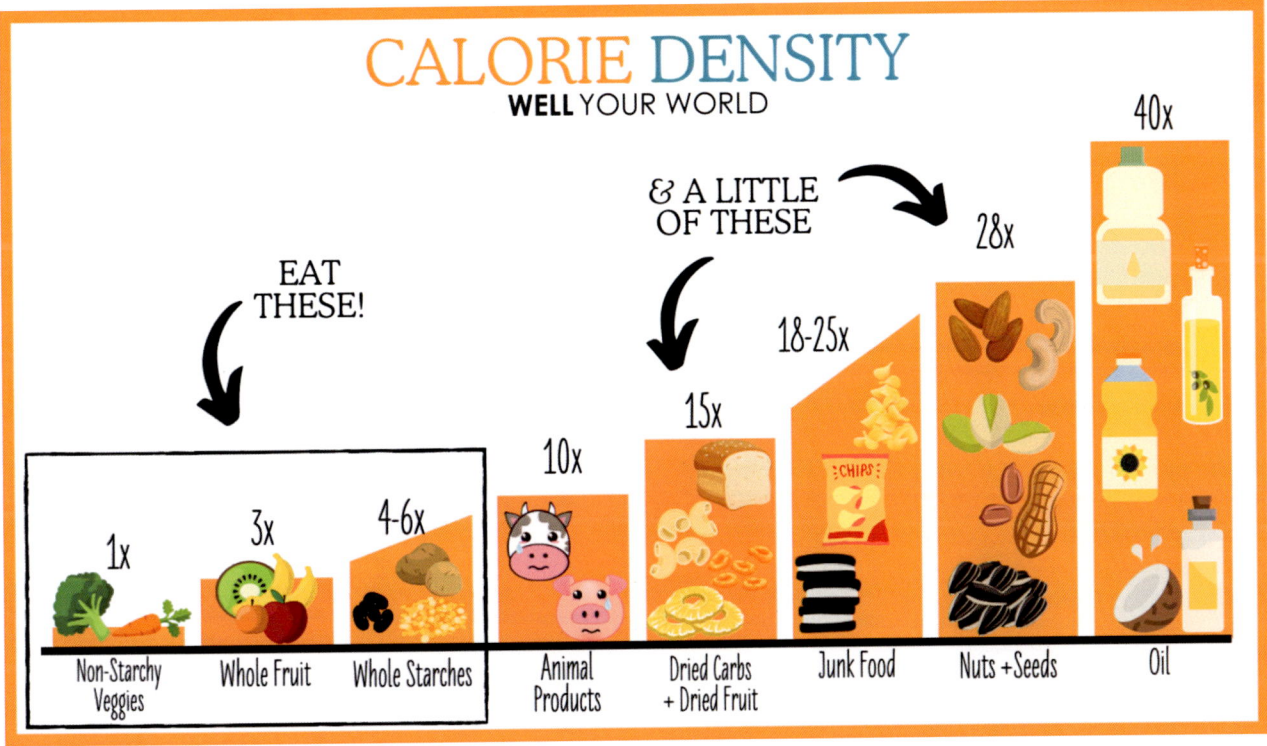

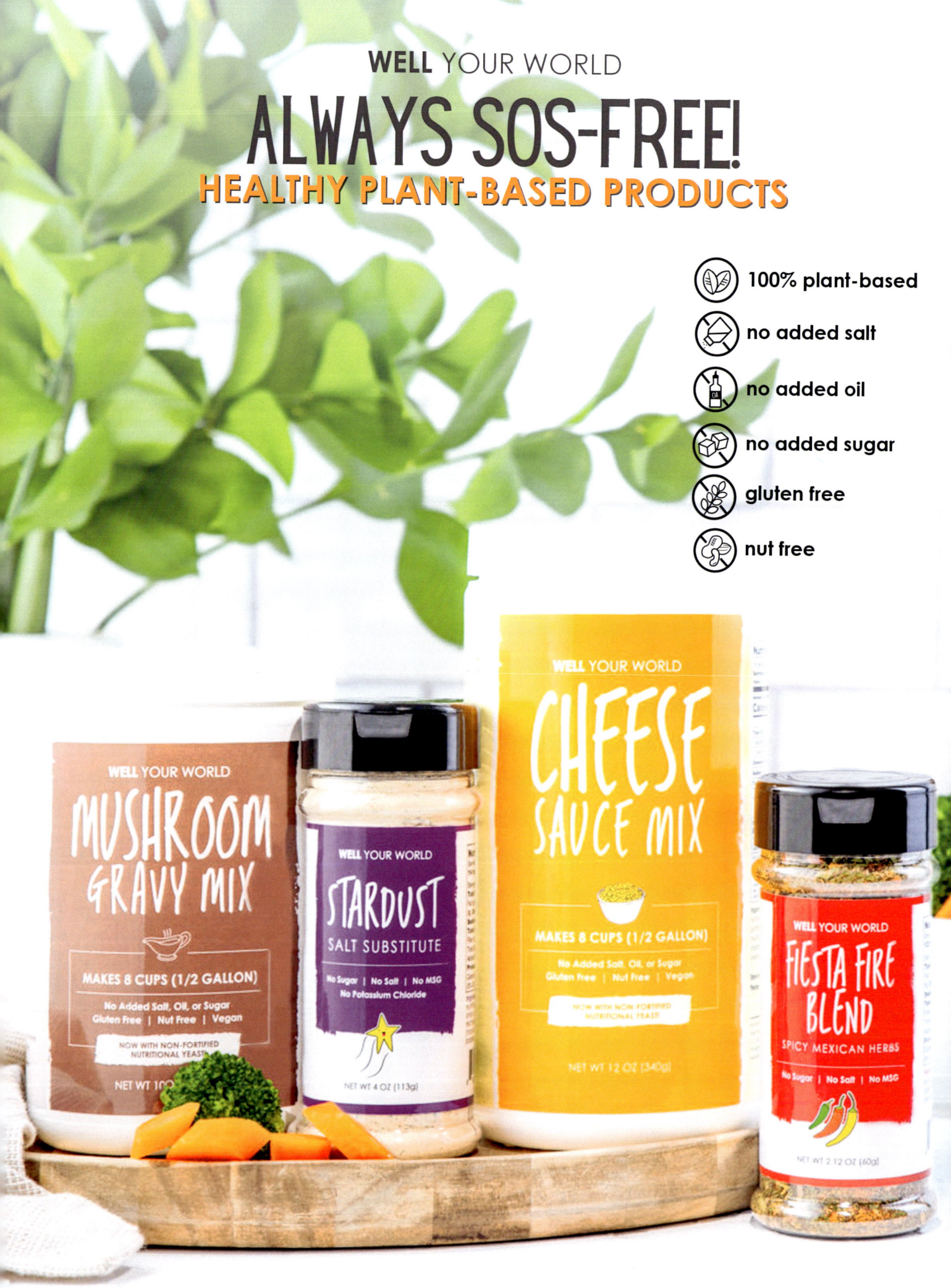

# WHY SOS-FREE?

Virtually all of the recipes on our YouTube channel, in our live cooking show, as well as all of our food products are free of salt, oil, and sugar (SOS).

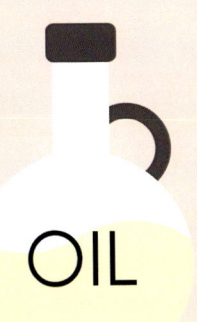

Oil is without question the worst offender in terms of calorie density. It is highly processed, void of any notable nutrient content, and 100% fat. Oil is 40x richer than broccoli! Plus, it is responsible for many adverse health problems such as obesity, heart disease, and type 2 diabetes.

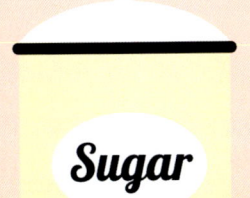

Sugar generally isn't as bad as oil in terms of detrimental health effects, but it is still very calorie dense, at 1,800 calories per pound. Higher calorie density = richer flavor = harder to stop eating. Before you know it, you've just eaten a bunch of useless calories.

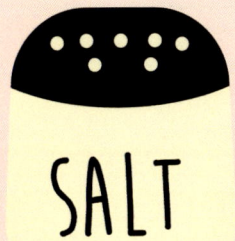

Salt is tricky because it doesn't have any calories. However, it can still hijack your taste buds and cause you to eat more than you otherwise would have. Many people avoid salt for other health reasons as well, such as hypertension or joint pain.

# FAQ'S

## HOW MANY SERVINGS DO YOUR RECIPES MAKE?

Honestly, we have no idea. We just don't think of it this way.

A "serving" is so personal to the individual. Some people have smaller appetites and some people can eat a large volume. Some people eat more frequently during the day and some people eat far less. "Servings" were created for people who count calories, and that is definitely not a sustainable way of eating. Instead of trying to limit your portion size, why not choose ingredients with lower calorie density instead?

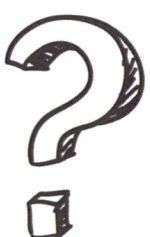

## CAN I FREEZE THE LEFTOVERS?

We get this question a lot and while the answer is usually yes, we always wonder WHY you would freeze the leftovers. If you make a meal that lasts several lunches the whole next week, that sounds like a win to us! Repeating meals or having leftovers in the fridge is not a bad thing. There is nothing wrong with freezing, but it does add a couple steps to your overall meal-prep process.

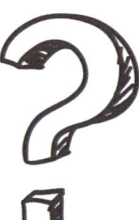

## I DONT LIKE A CERTAIN SPICE, CAN I REPLACE IT?

If you don't like ANYTHING in a recipe, we strongly encourage you to replace or omit it. Something like an Indian spice blend can also be replaced with a Mexican or Italian spice blend to give the recipe a whole new flavor. Feel free to experiment in the kitchen! Most of our recipes are very forgiving, so have fun and discover what you like!

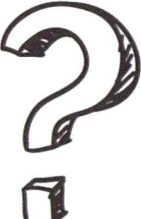

## I MADE A DISH AND DONT LIKE IT, HOW CAN I DOCTOR IT UP?

Our honest answer to this is to cut your losses and remove this dish from your rotation. You can try doctoring up a recipe you don't love with hot sauce, additional spices, or even air-frying it depending on the dish, but don't be afraid to toss the occasional meal you just don't love. It probably happens so infrequently that it's not going to matter in the grand scheme of things. And the best part is you learned something about your own tastes.

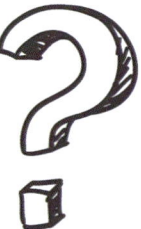

## I DONT HAVE TIME TO MAKE EVEN THE FASTEST MEAL, WHAT DO I DO?

You're in luck! We have an entire lineup of healthy products that we created to get you in and out of the kitchen even faster. You can whip up mac and cheese, banana pancakes, pasta, and salads with our time-saving products that are plant-based and salt, oil, and sugar free.

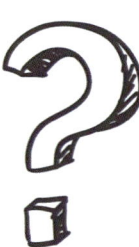

# TABLE OF CONTENTS

## APPS, SAMMIES, & WRAPS

| | |
|---|---|
| Simple Chickpea Bruschetta | 23 |
| Chickpea Lettuce Cups | 25 |
| Hearty-Choke Sandwich | 27 |
| Smashed Chickpea Avocado Wrap | 29 |
| McReebs Burger Wrap | 31 |
| BBQ Summer Wrap | 33 |
| MmmBLT Wrap | 35 |
| Sushirito | 37 |

## SOUPS & STEWS

| | |
|---|---|
| World's Fastest Lentil Stew | 39 |
| Mexican Fiesta Chili | 41 |
| Potato Corn Chowder | 43 |
| Indian Chili | 45 |

## MEALS

| | |
|---|---|
| Peanut Ramen Bowl | 47 |
| Mexican Buddha Bowl | 49 |

## MEALS CONT.

| | |
|---|---|
| One Pot Eggplant Delight | 51 |
| Simple Seasoned Lentils | 53 |
| Speedy Black-Eyed Peas & Greens | 55 |
| Stovetop Wowatouille | 57 |
| Curried Potato Stew | 59 |
| Pasta Carbonara | 61 |
| Teriyaki Stir Fry | 63 |
| Veggie Fajitas | 65 |
| Reebs' Riced Cauliflower | 67 |
| Creamy Butter Beans | 69 |
| Spaghetti Orz-Os | 71 |
| Microwaved Fried Rice | 73 |
| Sweet Potato Black Bean Bowl | 75 |
| Stuffed Sweet Potatoes | 77 |
| African Peanut Stew | 79 |
| Mushroom Stroganoff | 81 |
| Mexican Microwaved Rice | 83 |
| Stuffed Pepper Bowl | 85 |

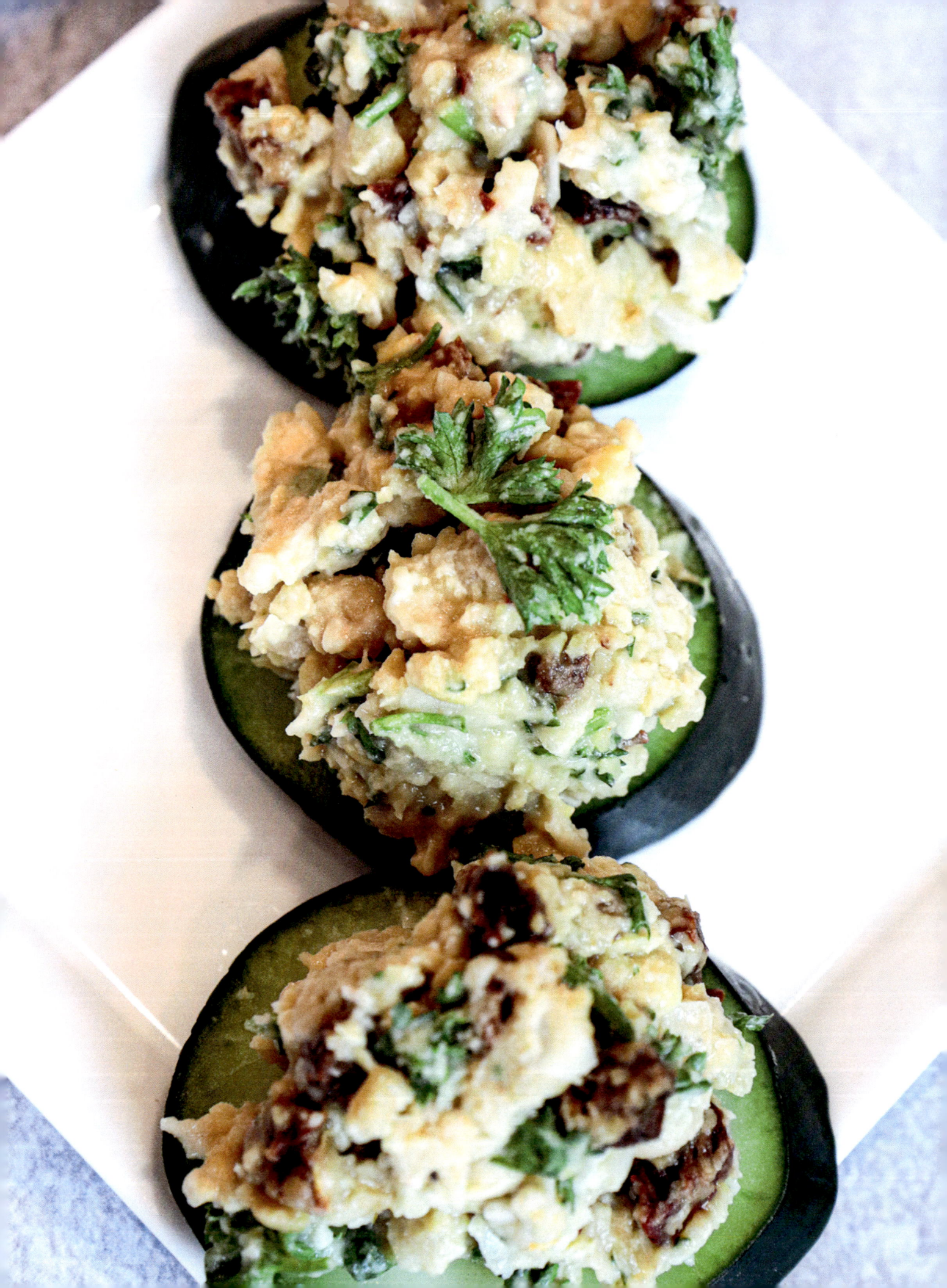

# SIMPLE CHICKPEA BRUSCHETTA

This recipe requires no heat, so it is great to make during the summer months when it's just too hot to cook! Enjoy on carrot chips, cucumber chips, a bed of greens, or make a tasty wrap.

## INGREDIENTS

- 1 15 oz. can chickpeas, drained and rinsed
- 1 tablespoon minced garlic
- 1/4 teaspoon crushed red pepper (optional)
- 2 tablespoons tahini
- 1 lemon, juiced
- 1 handful parsley, chopped
- 1/4 cup sun dried tomatoes, chopped

### Serve With
- whole grain bread or lavash, toasted
- cucumber chips
- carrot chips
- a bed of greens

## METHOD

Add the chickpeas, garlic, and crushed red pepper to a mixing bowl and mash into a coarse texture with a potato masher or fork.

Next, add the remaining ingredients to the bowl and mix well.

Enjoy on toast or whole wheat lavash, a bed of lettuce, with carrot chips, cucumber chips, crackers, and so much more! Make it a wrap, make it a dip, make it a spread, or make it a topper!

---

Note: Instead of sun-dried tomatoes, you can also try this with chopped cherry tomatoes for a juicier bite.

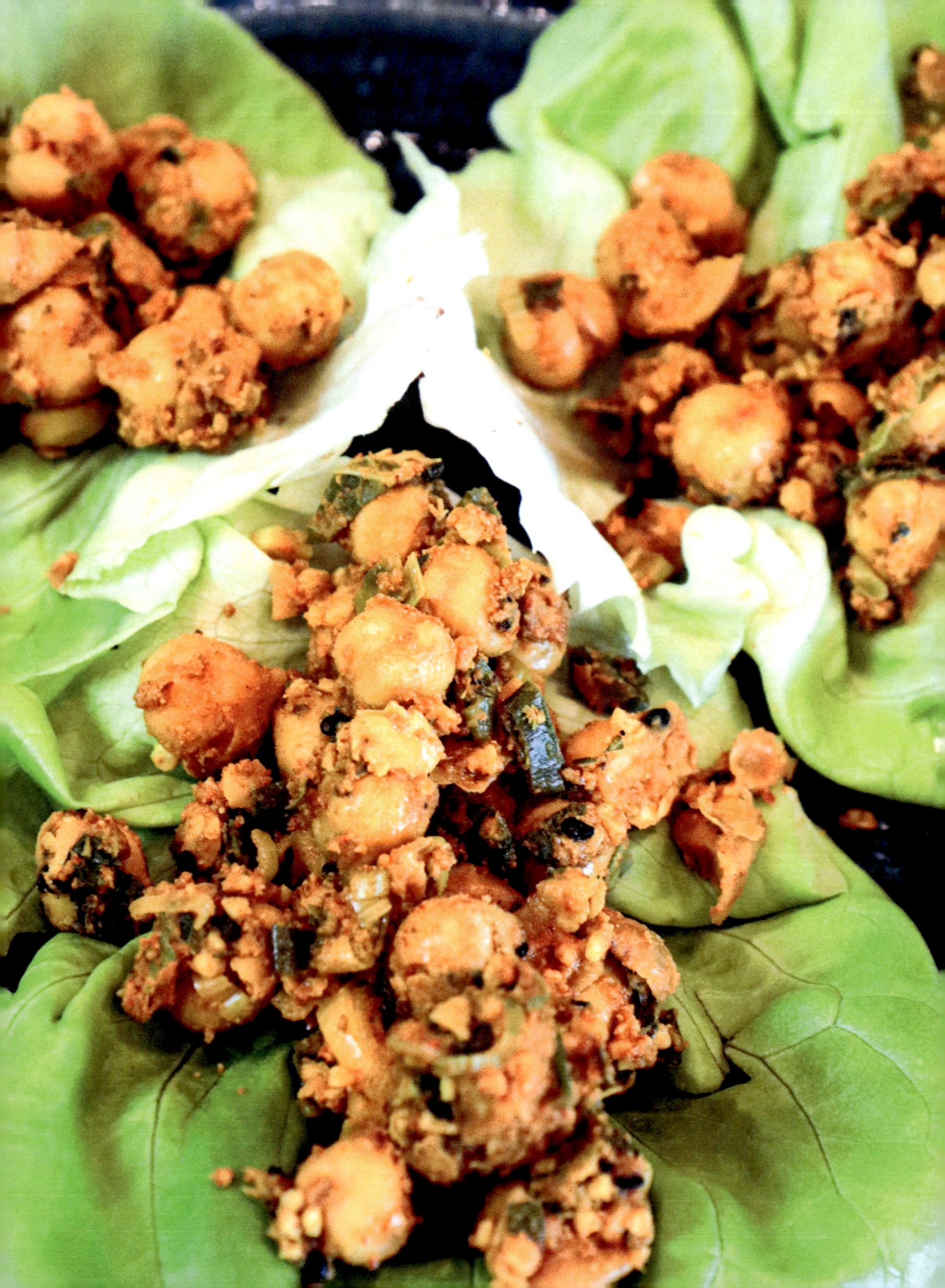

# CHICKPEA LETTUCE CUPS

Step aside P.F. Chang's! These lettuce wraps put theirs to shame!
Use this recipe as a blank canvas to add a Latin, Italian, Cajun, or Caribbean spin.

## INGREDIENTS

- 1    15 oz. can chickpeas, drained and rinsed
- 1    teaspoon ground turmeric
- 1    teaspoon ground cumin
- 1    teaspoon curry powder
- 1/2    teaspoon chili powder
- 1    green onion, chopped
- 3    garlic cloves, minced
- 6-8    mint leaves, chopped
- 1    tablespoon sesame seeds

   lettuce, to serve
   avocado, to serve

## METHOD

Heat up a skillet on the stove and add a few tablespoons of water along with the chickpeas, turmeric, cumin, curry, and chili powder. Stir together to coat the chickpeas.

Once the water has mostly cooked off, add the green onion, garlic, mint, and sesame seeds and stir for about a minute.

To serve, spoon some of the chickpea mixture onto the lettuce cups and top with avocado. Or serve them on a salad to make it starchy and filling. Enjoy!

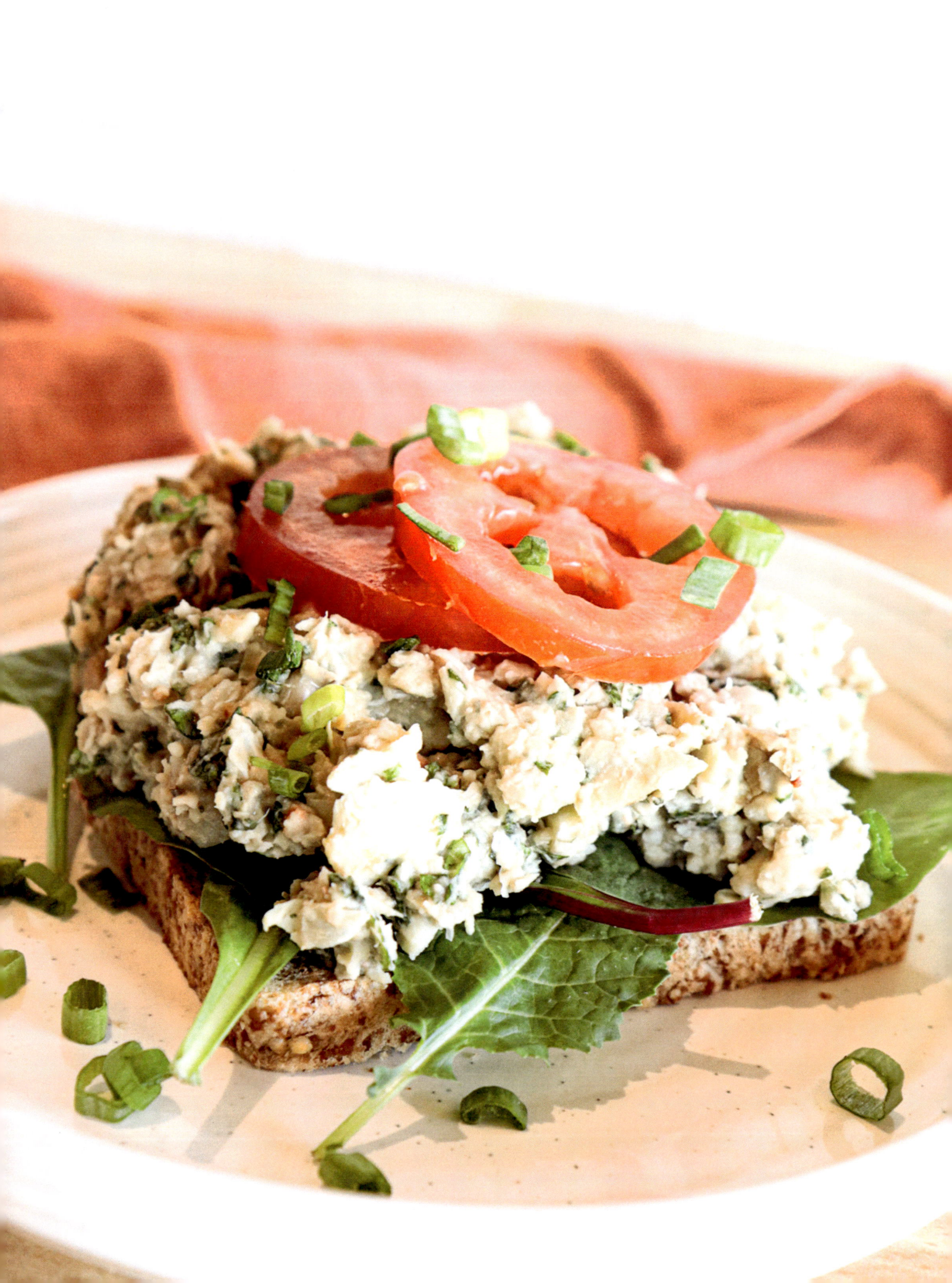

# HEARTY-CHOKE SANDWICH

I'm in love with artichokes and basil, and this recipe has both. Don't just make sandwiches with this recipe, use it as a spread for toast and wraps or even as a dip!

## INGREDIENTS

- 8 oz. frozen/canned artichoke hearts, thawed
- 1 15 oz. can white beans, drained and rinsed
- 3 garlic cloves, minced
- 1 handful fresh basil
- 1/2 lemon, juiced
- 1 tablespoon tahini (optional)
- 1-2 teaspoons favorite no-salt seasoning

### Serve With
- whole grain bread or lavash, toasted/warmed
- fresh spinach or lettuce
- sliced red or green onion
- sliced tomato
- black pepper

## METHOD

Add all of the ingredients to a food processor and pulse a few times. Wipe down the sides and pulse again until it reaches a slightly creamy but coarse texture.

Spread the mixture on the toast and add your favorite sandwich toppings. Enjoy!

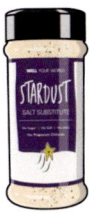

**Try our delicious Stardust Salt Substitute in this dish!**

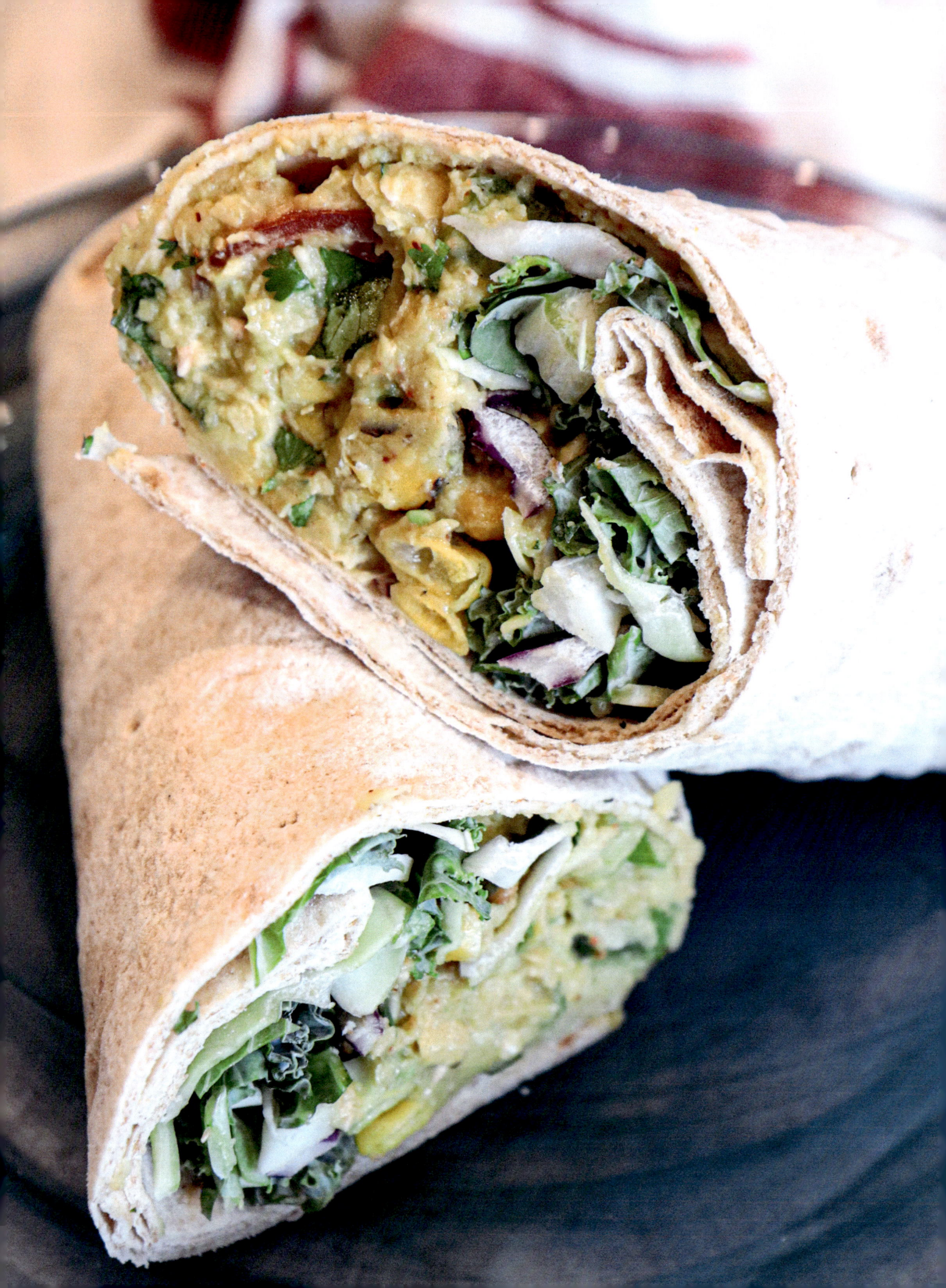

# SMASHED CHICKPEA AVOCADO WRAP

This recipe is even better than guac because of all the ingredients that make it so filling and flavorful! You can use this on just about anything, but our favorite way is to make wraps with whole wheat lavash, cruciferous crunch, and corn.

## INGREDIENTS

**Dip**
- 2 15 oz. cans chickpeas, drained and rinsed
- 1-2 avocados
- 1 jalapeño, seeded and diced
- 3 green onions, sliced
- 1 pint cherry tomatoes, halved
- 2 garlic cloves, minced
- 2 limes, juiced
- 1/4 cup fresh cilantro, chopped

**Wrap**
- whole wheat lavash
- lettuce or Trader Joe's Cruciferous Crunch
- sliced red onion
- char-roasted corn

## METHOD

To make the dip, add the chickpeas to a large mixing bowl and use a potato masher to smash them into a coarse, chunky texture.

Toss in the avocado and continue mashing to mix it together. Add the rest of the dip ingredients and stir to combine.

Make a wrap by adding the dip to a whole wheat lavash or tortilla and add all of the fixings you like!

Note: You can also eat this as a dip with carrot chips and cucumbers, as a salad topper, or with crackers as an appetizer!

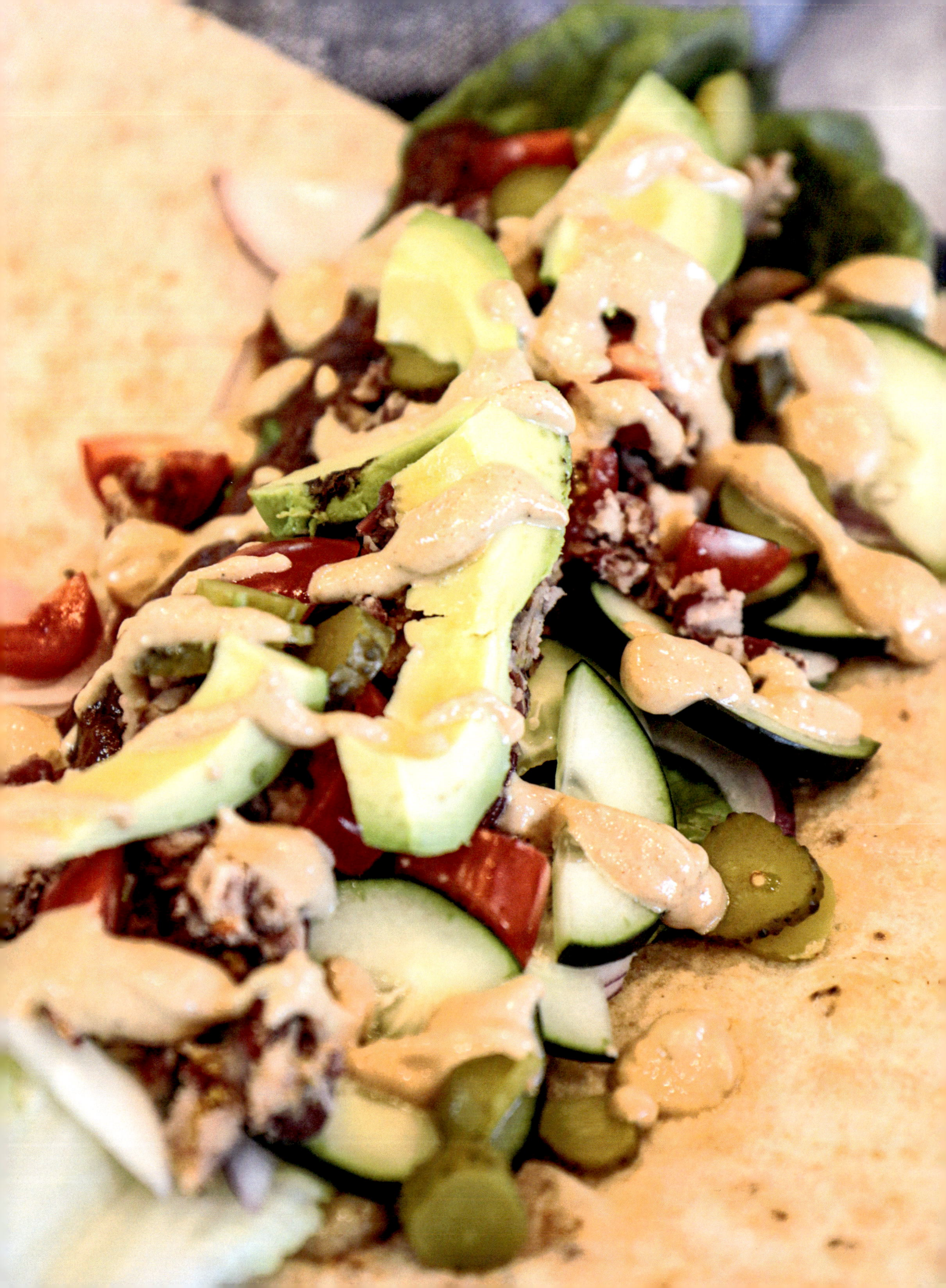

# MCREEBS BURGER WRAP

Don't waste time preparing a veggie burger from scratch, enjoy all the flavors of a veggie burger in this simple and satisfying wrap!

## INGREDIENTS

### McReebs Secret Sauce
- 1/2 cup raw cashews
- 1/2 cup water
- 1/4 cup ketchup
- 1 tablespoon nutritional yeast
- 1 teaspoon dijon or yellow mustard
- 1/2 teaspoon paprika
- 1 green onion
- 1 small lemon, juiced

### Burger Mash
- 1 15 oz. can kidney beans, drained and rinsed
- 1 tablespoon of your favorite spice blend

### Wrap
- whole wheat lavash
- romaine lettuce
- cherry tomatoes, quartered
- red onion, thinly sliced
- cucumbers, thinly sliced
- pickles, chopped
- avocado
- McReebs Secret Sauce

## METHOD

To prepare the McReebs Secret Sauce, add all of the ingredients to a high-speed blender and blend until smooth.

To prepare the Burger Mash, mash the kidney beans together with your favorite no-salt spice blend (we love WYW Galaxy Dust) in a small bowl using a potato masher or a fork.

To assemble the wrap, lay out the whole wheat lavash, add some mashed kidney beans along with all of the other wrap ingredients, drizzle on the McReebs sauce, roll it up, cut the wrap in half and enjoy! We love it dipped in a side of even more McReebs Sauce.

Note: This also makes a delicious salad. Add some air-fried french fries, we dare you!

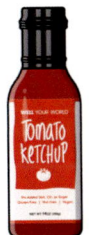

Try our delicious Tomato Ketchup in this viral McReebs Sauce! You'll love it!

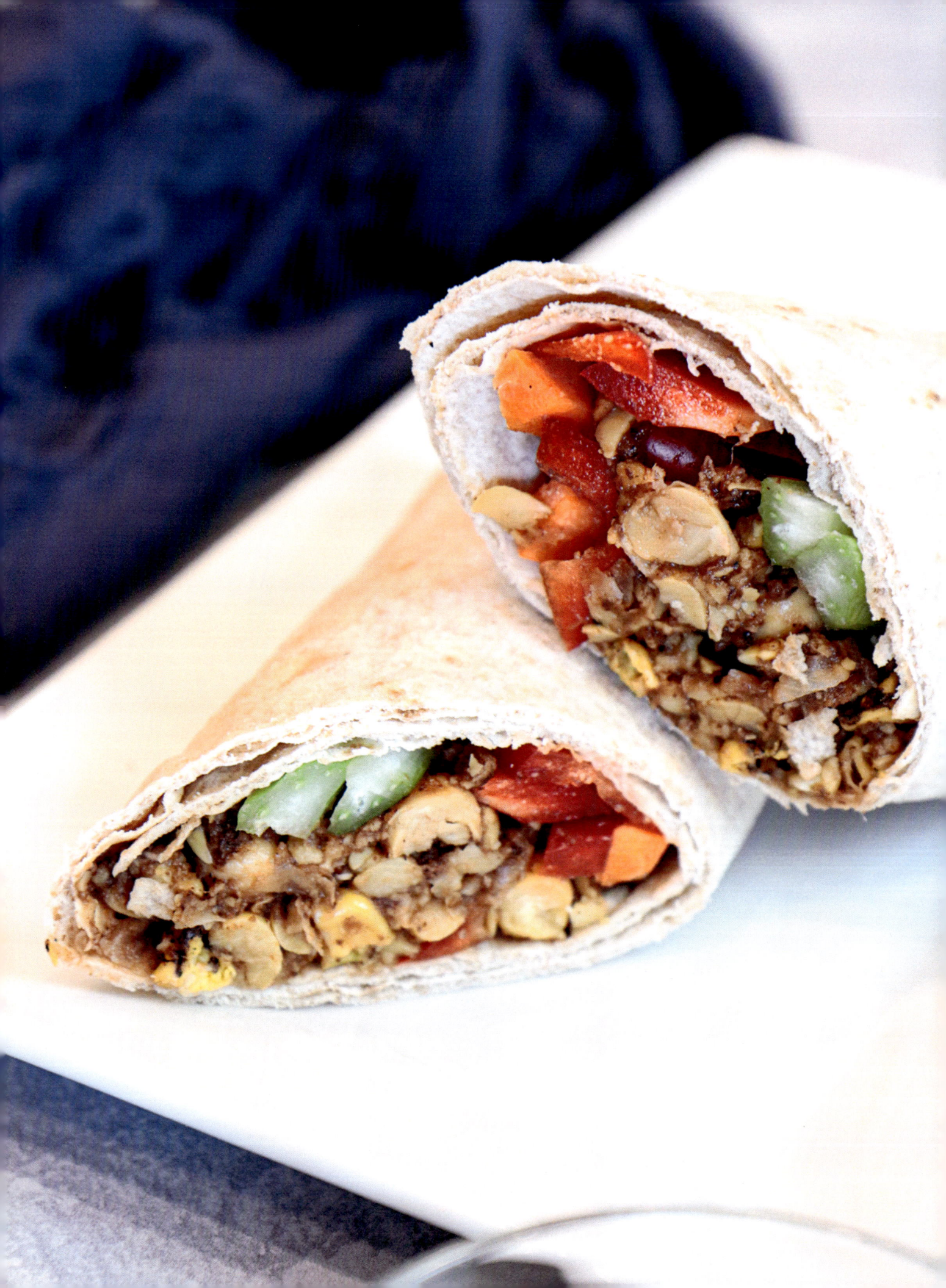

# BBQ SUMMER WRAP

The combination of flavors in this wrap will definitely remind you of summertime! From BBQ sauce, to corn, cucumber, and bell pepper, this wrap is full of nostalgic, summer delight.

## INGREDIENTS

### BBQ Sauce
- 2 tablespoons tomato paste
- 2 tablespoons apple cider vinegar
- 1/2 teaspoon garlic powder
- 1/2 teaspoon onion powder
- 1/8 teaspoon ground cinnamon
- 2 whole cloves
- 1/4 teaspoon white pepper
- 5 deglet dates
- 1 teaspoon paprika
- 1 teaspoon mustard
- 1/4 teaspoon liquid smoke
- 2/3 cup water
- 1/8 teaspoon celery seed

### Chickpea Filling
- 1 15 oz. can chickpeas, drained and rinsed
- 1/2 cup frozen fire roasted corn, thawed
- 1/2 cup BBQ sauce

### Wrap Ingredients
- Trader Joe's whole wheat lavash or whole grain bread
- Chickpea Filling
- 1-2 ribs celery, sliced thin
- 1 red bell pepper, sliced thin
- 1 carrot, sliced thin
- 1/2 cucumber, sliced thin
- 1 avocado, sliced

## METHOD

To make the BBQ sauce, add all of the ingredients to a high-speed blender or bullet blender and blend until smooth. If you prefer a sweeter flavor, blend in a few extra dates or date powder.

In a mixing bowl, add the chickpeas, corn, and BBQ sauce. Mash into a coarse texture with a potato masher.

Lay out the whole wheat lavash, add some chickpea filling along with as much of the other wrap ingredients as you like, roll it up, and cut the wrap in half.

Enjoy this no-heat Summer recipe! This will yield at least a couple wraps.

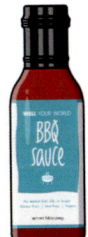

**Simplify this recipe by using our healthy bottled BBQ Sauce!**

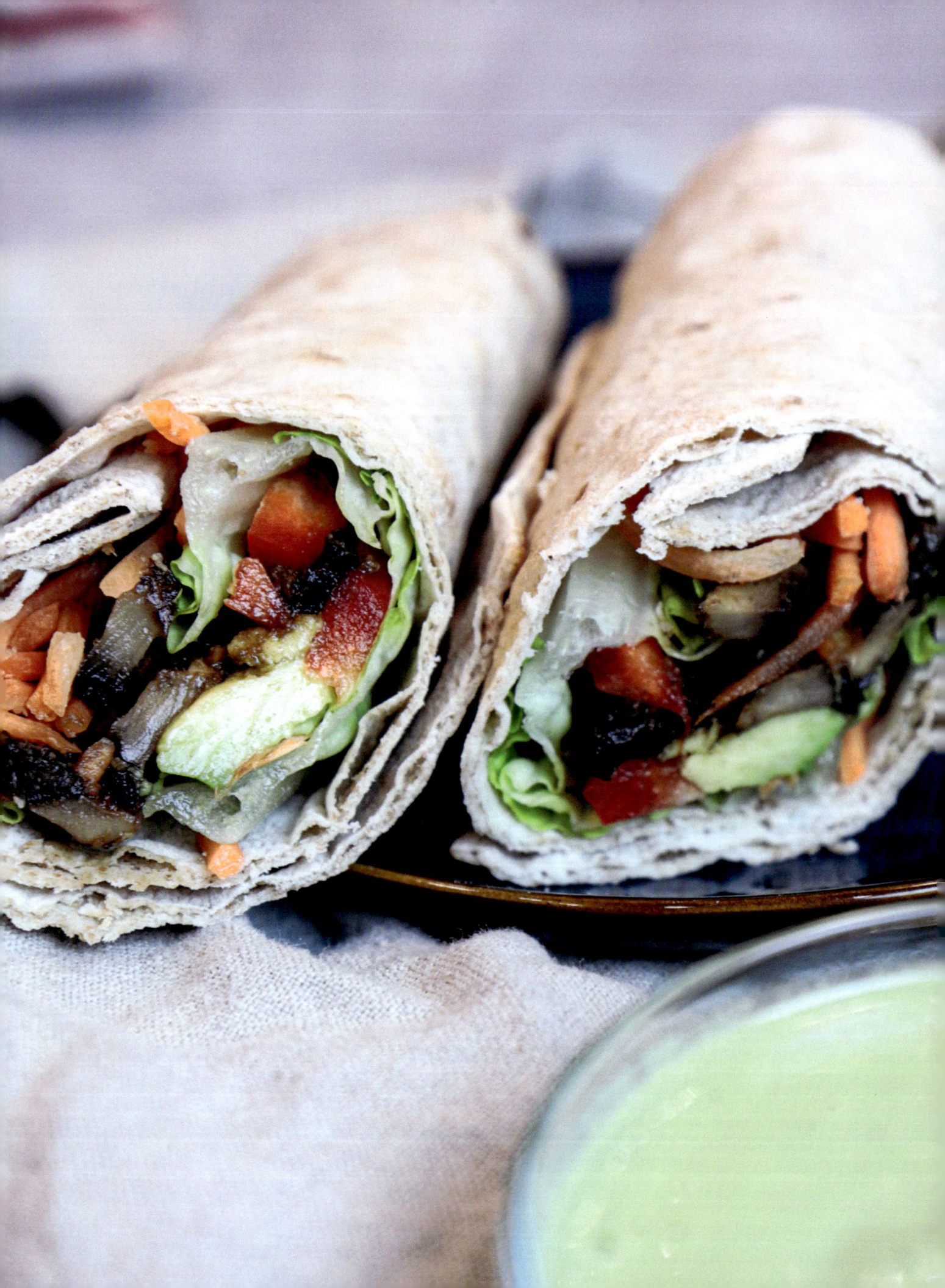

# MMMBLT WRAP

This wrap has all of the fixings of a BLT and then some! You are definitely going to love the creamy jalapeño and dill sauce...I mean Dillapeño Sauce.

## INGREDIENTS

### Mushroom Bacon
- 1/2 cup veggie broth
- 1/2 teaspoon liquid smoke
- 2 tablespoons balsamic vinegar
- 1 teaspoon garlic powder
- 1 teaspoon onion powder
- 1 teaspoon paprika
- 3-4 portobello mushrooms, sliced

### Dillapeño Sauce
- 1/4 cup tahini
- 1-2 tablespoons fresh chopped dill
- 1 jalapeño, seeds removed
- 1 lime, juiced
- 1-2 deglet dates
- 2 garlic cloves
- 1+ tablespoons water, as needed
- black pepper, to taste

### Wrap
- Trader Joe's Whole Wheat Lavash or whole grain bread
- romaine or butter lettuce
- cherry tomatoes, quartered
- red bell pepper, sliced
- cucumbers, sliced
- carrots, shredded
- mushroom bacon
- Dillapeño Sauce

## METHOD

To prepare the mushroom bacon, add all of the ingredients to a saucepan and sauté over medium-high heat, stirring occasionally. Continue to sauté until the mushrooms have softened to your liking and most of the liquid has cooked off. Set aside.

To prepare the Dillapeño Sauce, add all of the ingredients to a high-speed blender, reserving about 1/2 the dill, and blend until smooth. Add the remaining dill and pulse a few times to leave some green dill texture in the sauce.

To prepare the wrap, lay out the whole wheat lavash, add some mushrooms along with all of the other wrap ingredients. Drizzle on the Dillapeño Sauce, roll it up, cut in half and enjoy!

Save some Dillapeño Sauce for dipping!

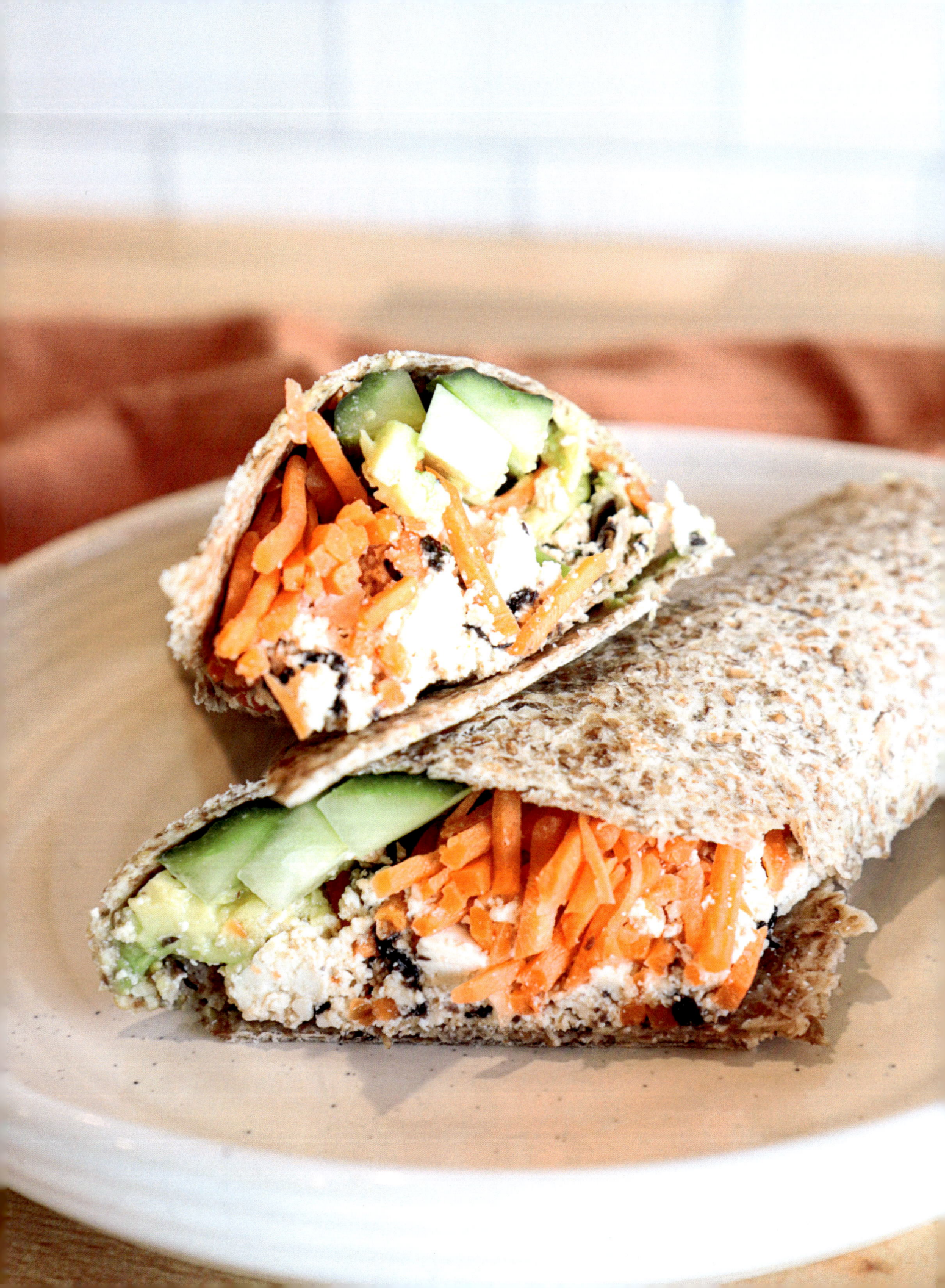

# SUSHIRRITO

Love the flavor of sushi, but rolling them is a pain? Then this recipe is for you! Enjoy the flavors of sushi wrapped into a simple burrito.

## INGREDIENTS

### Tofu Mix

| | |
|---|---|
| 1/2 | 14-16 oz. extra firm block tofu |
| 1 | teaspoon garlic powder |
| 1 | teaspoon onion powder |
| 1 | teaspoon sesame seeds |
| 1 | teaspoon soy sauce (optional) |
| 1 | teaspoon rice vinegar |
| 1/2-1 | teaspoon Sriracha |
| 1 | sheet nori, chopped |
| 1 | green onion, sliced |

### Sushi Burrito

- whole wheat lavash or Ezekiel tortilla
- cooked rice
- avocado
- carrot
- cucumber
- Tofu Mix

## METHOD

To prepare the Tofu Mix, crumble the tofu into a large mixing bowl using your hands. Add the remaining ingredients and toss to combine. If chopping the nori is challenging, you can use a pair of sheers to cut it up as well.

To prepare the Sushi Burrito, lay out the wrap, add some rice, and press flat. Add all of the other burrito ingredients, roll it up, cut in half, and enjoy!

Note: You can make this recipe into a sushi bowl too!

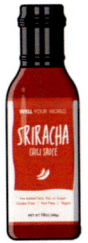

Add a touch of heat with our deliciously spicy Sriracha sauce.

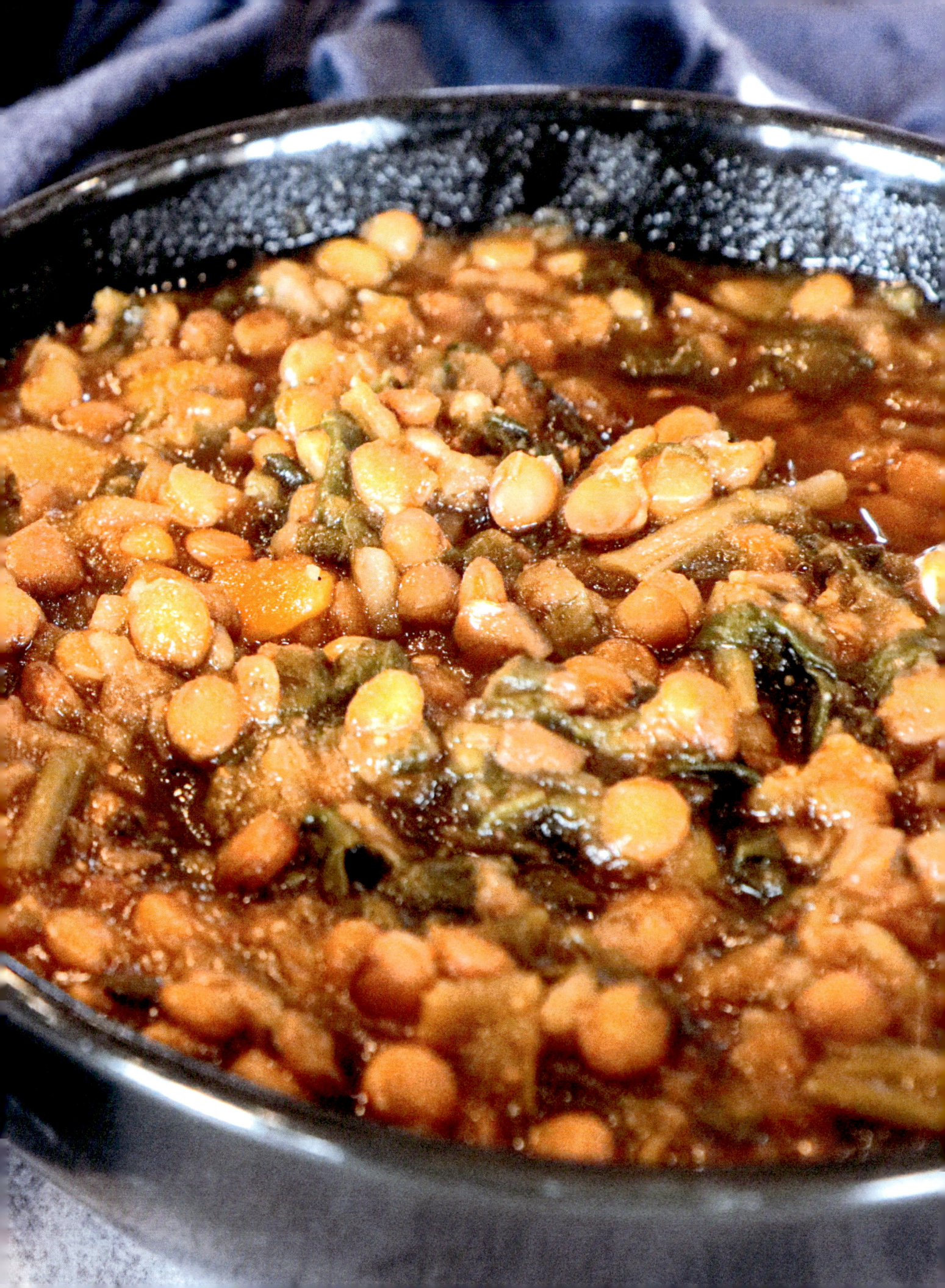

# WORLD'S FASTEST LENTIL STEW

Nothing beats a no-chop, one pot meal! Simply toss all of the ingredients into a pot and heat it up. Use any of your favorite spice blends to switch it up from time to time.

## INGREDIENTS

### Stew
- 12 cups water or veggie broth
- 3 cups brown lentils, cooked (or 2 15 oz. cans)
- 1/2 cup dehydrated onion
- 4 tablespoons Berbere or favorite spice blend
- 2 1 lb. bags frozen chopped spinach
- 2 10-12 oz. bags chopped butternut squash
- 1 6 oz. can tomato paste

### Berbere Spice Blend
- 2 teaspoons paprika
- 2 teaspoons coriander
- 2 teaspoons ground ginger
- 2 teaspoons ground cumin
- 2 teaspoons garlic powder
- 1-2 teaspoons chili pepper
- 1 teaspoon ground fenugreek
- 1/2 teaspoon ground cardamom
- 1/8 teaspoon ground cloves

## METHOD

Add all of the ingredients to a large stock pot and bring to a boil. Reduce heat to medium and simmer for 5-10 minutes, stirring occasionally.

The Westbrae Natural canned no-salt lentils are great for this, or use pre-cooked lentils from the fridge!

The Berbere Spice Blend recipe will make the perfect amount needed for this recipe.

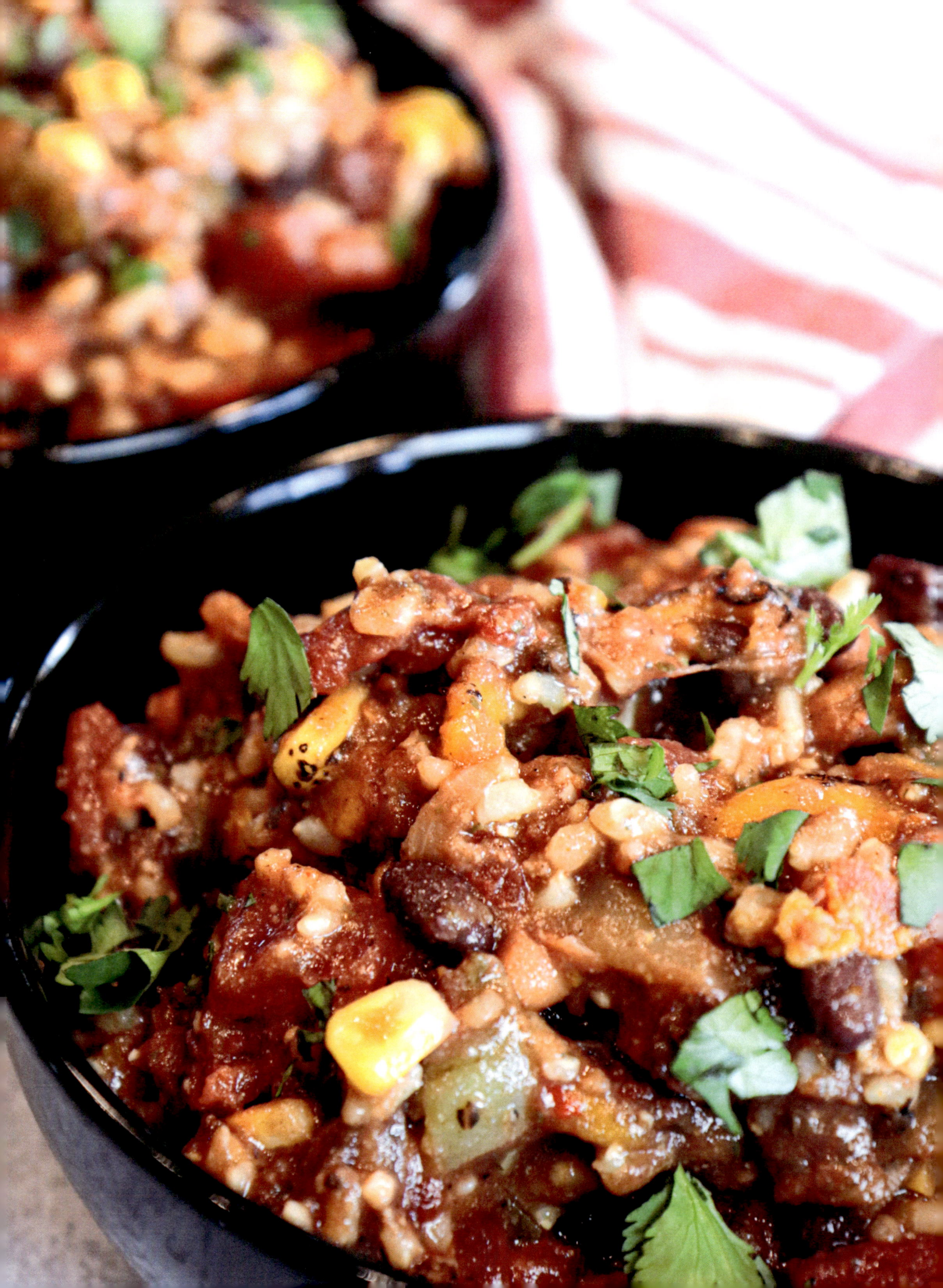

# MEXICAN FIESTA CHILI

This colorful Mexican chili brings together the delicious flavors of bell peppers, corn, and tangy tomatoes, all cooked in one pot for a satisfying meal that takes no time at all!

## INGREDIENTS

- 2 — 15 oz. cans diced tomatoes
- 1 — 15 oz. can tomato sauce
- 1 — 15 oz. can pinto beans, drained and rinsed
- 1 — 15 oz. can black beans, drained and rinsed
- 1 — 14-16 oz. bag frozen fire roasted peppers & onions
- 1/2 — 1 lb. bag frozen char roasted corn
- 1 — 10-12 oz. bag frozen brown rice
- 2 tablespoons nutritional yeast
- 1 tablespoon minced garlic
- 2 teaspoons dried oregano
- 1 teaspoon dried cilantro
- 1 teaspoon ground cumin
- 1 teaspoon chipotle powder
- 2 teaspoons date powder
- 1 teaspoon crushed red pepper (optional)

### Other Toppings

- squeeze of lime
- fresh chopped cilantro
- chopped black/green olives
- homemade chips
- corn tortillas

## METHOD

This is as simple as throwing all of the ingredients in a large soup pot and heating to a boil. Reduce the heat and let simmer for 5-10 minutes. Honestly, you could leave this on low all day long, and it will only get better.

Top with a squeeze of lime, fresh chopped cilantro, and/or chopped olives. I love eating this one with homemade chips or corn tortillas.

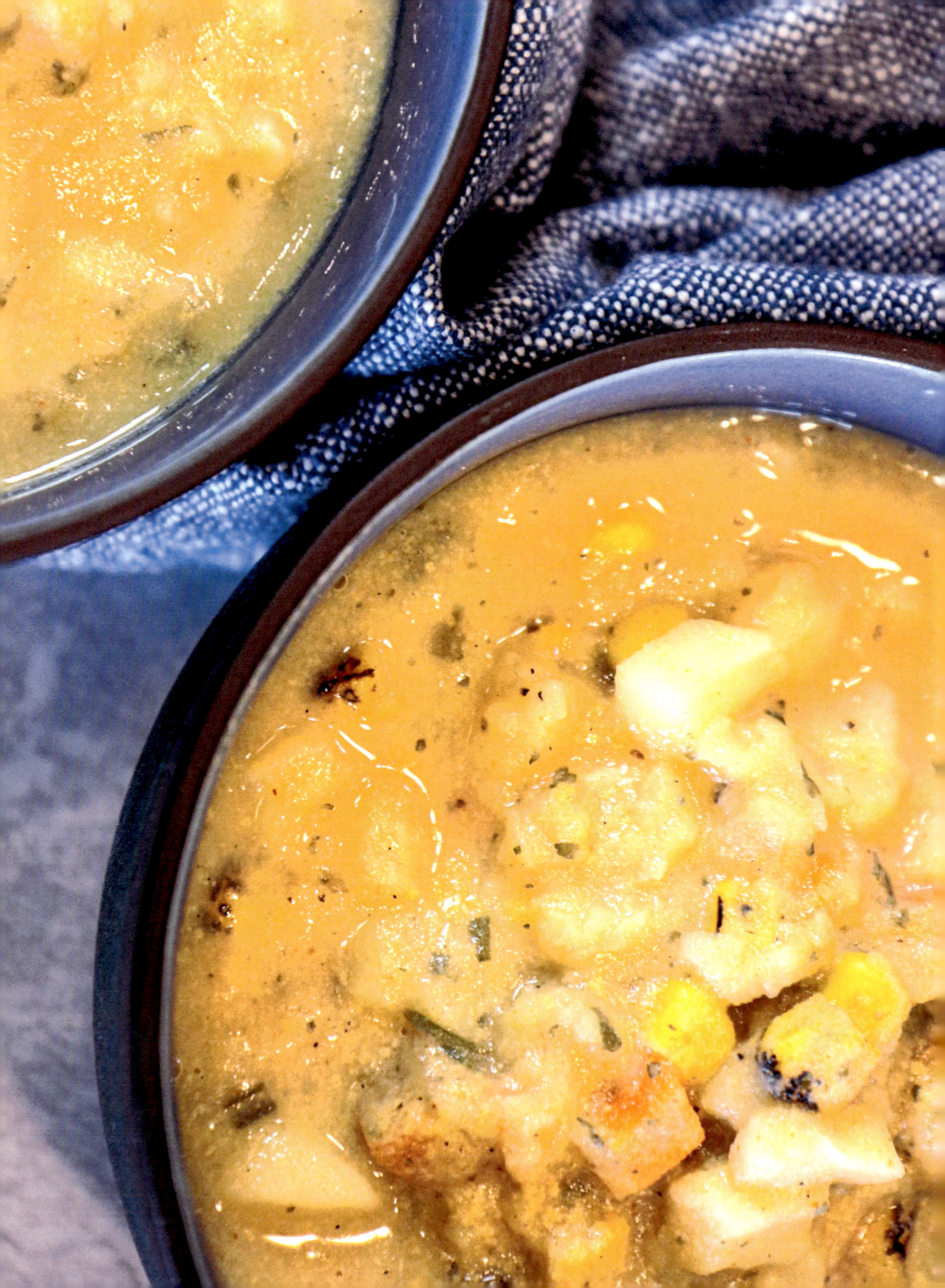

# POTATO CORN CHOWDER

This soup is so full of flavor that you will forget it took so little effort to whip up! Whether it's a super busy night or you just want a simple meal that will fill you up, you've turned to the right page! This is my favorite soup.

## INGREDIENTS

- 4 cups veggie broth
- 2 cups soy milk
- 1/4 cup nutritional yeast
- 2 teaspoons dried parsley
- 2 teaspoons dried chives
- 2 teaspoons garlic powder
- 1 teaspoon dried tarragon
- 1/2 teaspoon black pepper
- 1/2 teaspoon paprika
- 1 1 lb. bag frozen Potatoes O' Brien (cubed potatoes)
- 1 10-12 oz. bag frozen mirepoix mix (diced carrots, celery, and onion)
- 1 15 oz. can corn, drained and rinsed

## METHOD

Add all of the ingredients to a large soup pot, heat to a boil, reduce the heat and let simmer for a few minutes and enjoy!

You can cook this one for 5 minutes or 30 minutes, it doesn't matter. Feel free to swap any ingredient or flavoring with whatever you like. The point here is the process, so so simple!

Note: You can use canned corn or frozen corn interchangeably. We love using char-roasted frozen corn in this dish too!

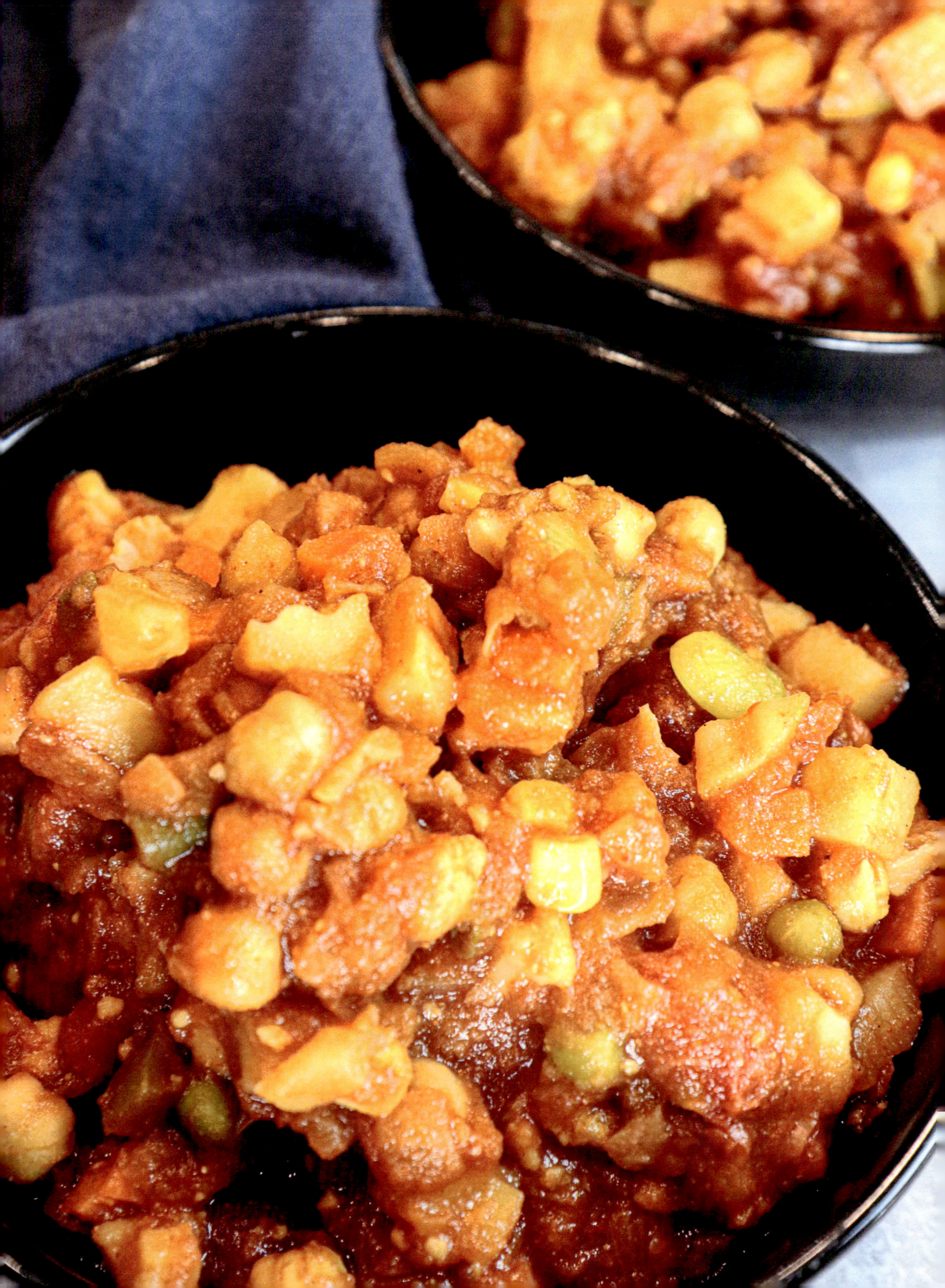

# INDIAN CHILI

With its vibrant colors and hearty texture, this dish is a perfect, speedy meal for those craving a nutritious and satisfying chili.

## INGREDIENTS

- 2   15 oz. cans tomato sauce
- 1   15 oz. can diced tomatoes
- 1   15 oz. can chickpeas, drained and rinsed
- 1   1 lb. bag frozen cauliflower florets
- 1   1 lb. bag frozen Potatoes O'Brien (cubed potatoes)
- 1   10-12 oz. bag frozen chopped onion
- 1 1/2   cups frozen mixed vegetables
- 1   tablespoon date powder
- 1   tablespoon minced garlic
- 1   tablespoon curry powder
- 1   tablespoon ground coriander
- 1   teaspoon ground cumin
- 1/2   teaspoon ground turmeric
- 1/2   teaspoon ground chili powder
- 1+   cups veggie broth

## METHOD

This is as simple as throwing all of the ingredients in a large soup pot and heating to a boil. Reduce the heat and let simmer for 5-10 minutes.

Adjust the veggie stock to reach your desired consistency. I like adding about a cup.

You could leave this on low all day long and it will only get better. Top with a squeeze of lime and fresh chopped cilantro, but it's delicious without as well.

Note: Save time and substitute the Indian herbs and spices (from garlic down to chili powder) with ~3 tablespoons of our WYW Indian Seasoning Blend, it is one of my favorites!

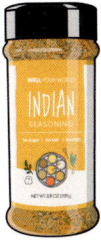

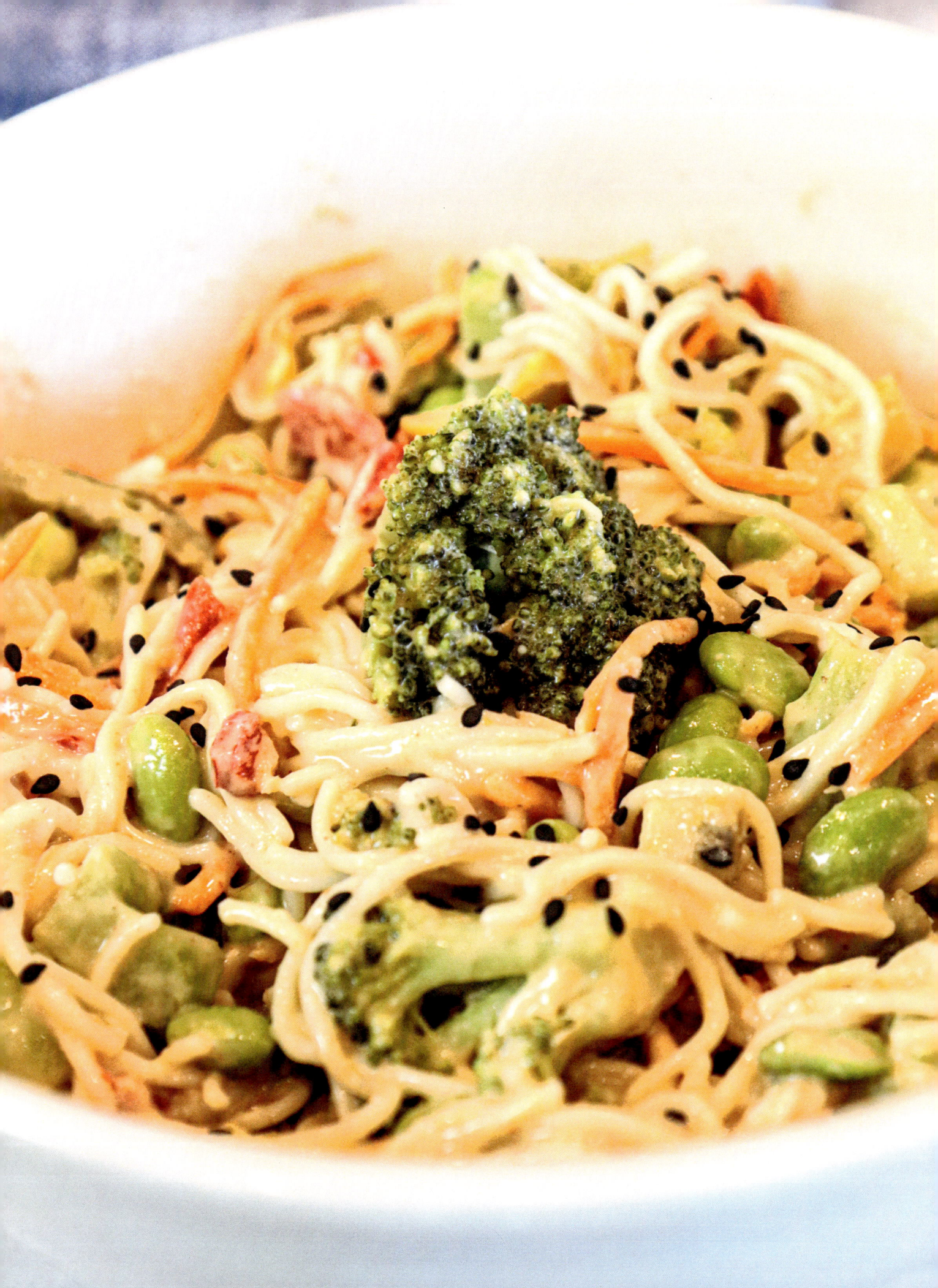

# PEANUT RAMEN BOWL

Once you make this recipe, you will be shocked at how easy it is to make restaurant quality ramen at home! Top with green onion and a sprinkle of sesame seeds for added crunch and flavor.

## INGREDIENTS

### Peanut Sauce

| | |
|---|---|
| 4-6 | tablespoons water |
| 1 | tablespoon lime juice |
| 1 | tablespoon rice vinegar |
| 1/3 | cup peanut butter |
| 1 | tablespoon soy sauce/tamari/miso (optional) |
| 2 | teaspoons date powder (or 2 deglet dates) |
| 1" | nub fresh ginger |
| 3 | garlic cloves |
| 1 | green onion |
| | crushed red pepper or Thai chilis, to taste |

### Ramen Bowl

- brown rice ramen
- frozen broccoli
- frozen bell peppers
- frozen shelled edamame
- Peanut Sauce
- broccoli slaw
- sliced green onion
- chopped cilantro
- sesame seeds

## METHOD

To prepare the Peanut Sauce, add all of the ingredients to a high-speed blender and blend until smooth. Set aside.

To prepare the Ramen Bowl, bring an oversized pot of water to a boil and throw in 2-3 ramen noodle blocks. Allow these to cook for about 5 minutes, using a fork to break them apart once they start to soften.

Then, add some frozen broccoli and shelled edamame to the water with the ramen noodles. Let this simmer a couple minutes longer, and then strain it out and transfer to a bowl. Toss with the Peanut Sauce and broccoli slaw. Sprinkle on some sliced green onion, cilantro, and sesame seeds. Enjoy!

Note: We love the Lotus Foods Brown Rice and Millet Ramen for this recipe!

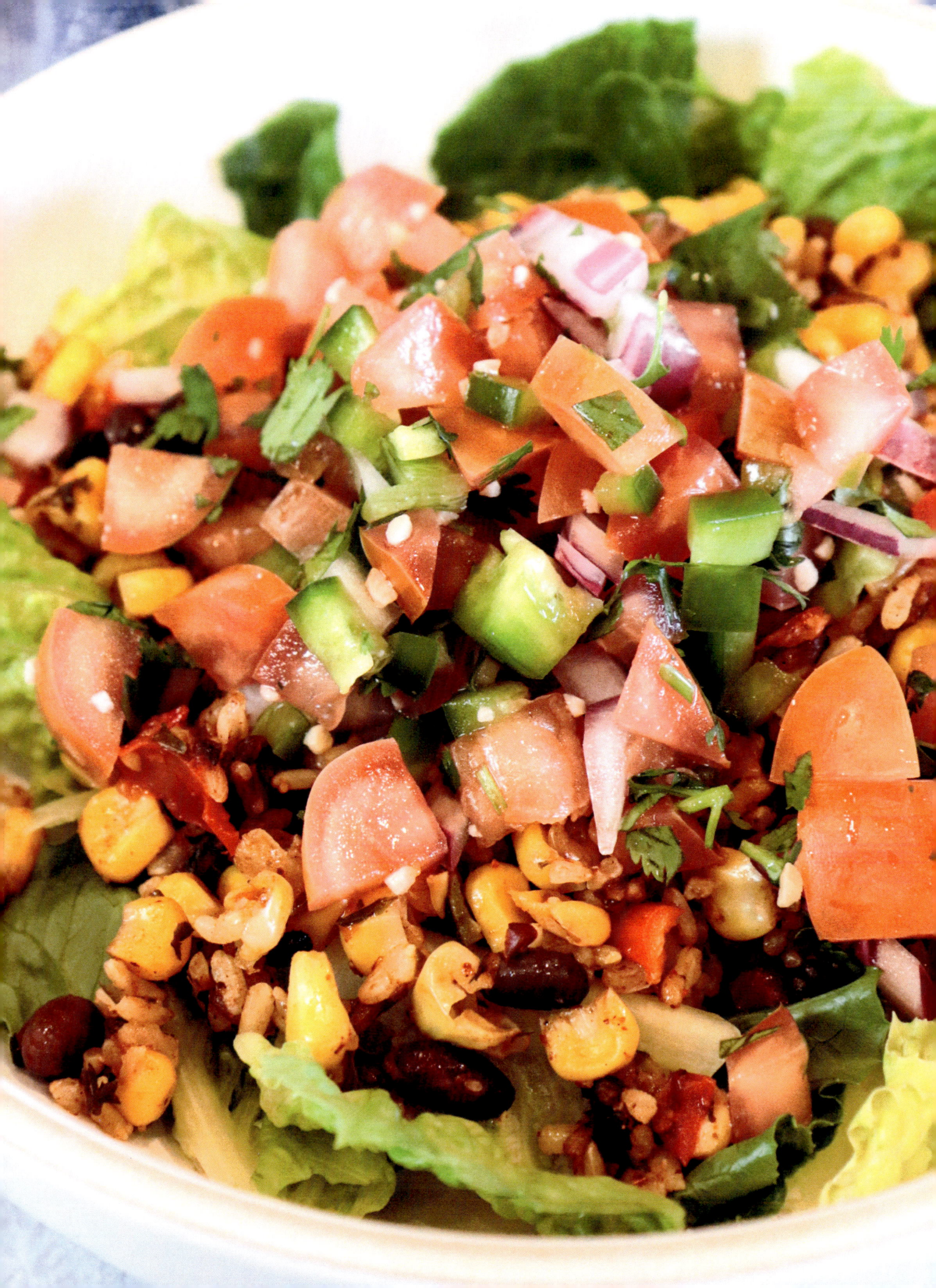

# MEXICAN BUDDHA BOWL

The steamer basket is your secret weapon in this recipe, turning basic freezer ingredients into a colorful Mexican-inspired meal in just minutes. No chopping required!

## INGREDIENTS

- 1   10-12 oz. bag frozen brown rice
- 1   14-16 oz. bag frozen "Southwest Veggies" (onions, bell peppers, corn, beans)
- 1-2 tablespoons no-salt Mexican taco seasoning like WYW Chili Lime or Fiesta Blend

### Additional Items
- romaine lettuce
- pico de gallo salsa
- chopped tomatoes
- sliced avocado
- cilantro
- fresh lime juice

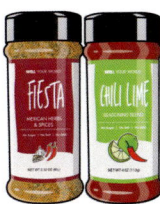

**Try our Chili Lime or Fiesta in this recipe!**

## METHOD

First, add the frozen rice to a steamer basket on the stove along with the bag of frozen Southwest veggies. The one we like includes black beans, corn, onion, and bell pepper all in one freezer bag. If you can't find that mix then you can build your own with a can of black beans and corn plus some frozen bell pepper and onions.

Add the seasoning right on top of the veggies, cover, and allow to steam for 5-10 minutes to heat through and soften the veggies. Then give it a stir, and it's ready!

To assemble, add a layer of chopped romaine lettuce to the bottom of a large plate or bowl and top with the steamed mix.

Feel free to top with any of the additional fresh items. We love to make a quick pico de gallo of chopped tomatoes, red onion, jalapeño, cilantro, lime juice, and some of our WYW Chili Lime seasoning. Sometimes we go as simple as just chopped tomatoes and avocado on top with the Chili Lime. Enjoy!

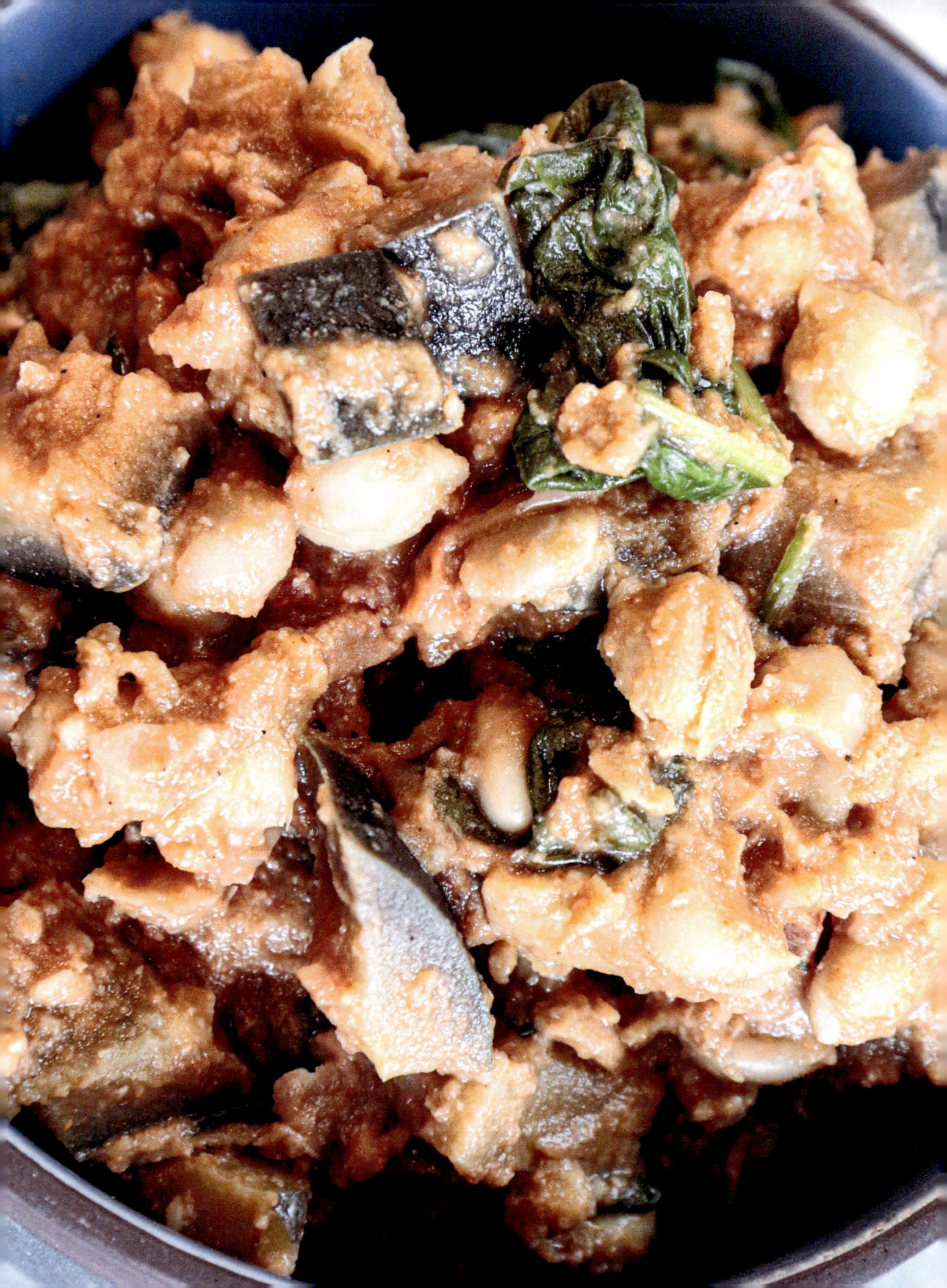

# ONE POT EGGPLANT BEAN DELIGHT

This hearty one-pot meal combines tender eggplant with two types of beans in a rich, spiced tomato sauce. One of our absolute favorites, it comes together in minutes and delivers incredible flavor with minimal effort!

## INGREDIENTS

- 1 eggplant, chopped into 1/4" cubes
- 2 teaspoons smoked paprika
- 1 teaspoon onion powder
- 1 teaspoon garlic powder
- 1 teaspoon date powder
- 1/2 teaspoon crushed red pepper (optional)
- 1 15 oz. can white beans, drained and rinsed
- 1 15 oz. can chickpeas, drained and rinsed
- 1 15 oz. can diced tomatoes
- 1 tablespoon tomato paste
- 1/2 lemon, juiced
- 1 tablespoon tahini (optional)
- 2 handfuls fresh spinach

## METHOD

Add the eggplant to a large pot and sauté over medium-high heat for 5-7 minutes until soft, adding veggie stock as needed to keep from sticking.

Add the paprika, onion powder, garlic powder, date powder, crushed red pepper, white beans, and chickpeas. Continue to sauté for a couple more minutes.

Stir in the diced tomatoes and tomato paste and heat back up to a simmer.

Add the lemon juice, tahini, and fresh spinach and mix well to cook the spinach for another minute or so.

Enjoy on its own or over your favorite starch like cooked lentils or rice.

Note: Feel free to use any leafy greens you have on hand! Fresh kale, collards, or frozen greens all work beautifully in this versatile dish.

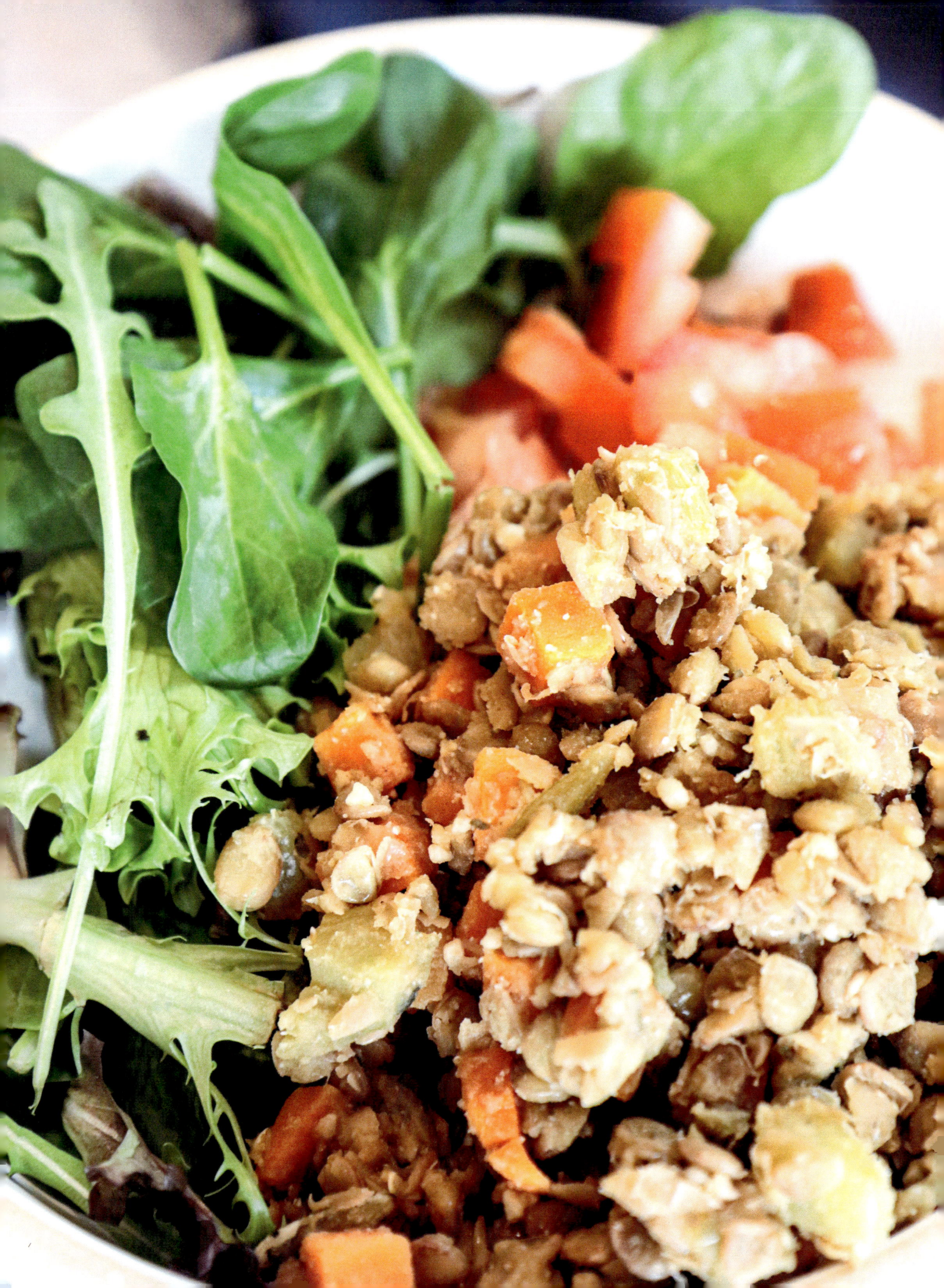

# SIMPLE SEASONED LENTILS

These savory, seasoned lentils transform pantry staples into a versatile meal base in minutes! Perfect on their own, over greens, or as a hearty side dish—this recipe delivers big flavor with minimal effort.

## INGREDIENTS

- 2    15 oz. cans lentils (or 3 cups cooked)
- 1    10-12 oz. bag frozen chopped onion
- 1    10-12 oz. bag frozen chopped bell peppers
- 2    teaspoons minced garlic
- 1-2 tablespoons no-salt seasoning
- 2    tablespoons pumpkin seeds (pepitas)
- 1    lime, juiced
- 1    handful fresh greens, chopped
- 1    tomato, chopped

## METHOD

Add the lentils, onion, bell peppers, and garlic to a large saucepan and sauté over medium-high heat for 5 minutes until tender, adding veggie broth as needed to keep from sticking.

Add your favorite no-salt seasoning along with the pepitas, and continue to sauté for another minute.

Squeeze on the lime and serve over a bed of greens topped with fresh chopped tomatoes. Enjoy!

Note: Switch it up with Italian seasoning and lemon juice instead of lime, then top with chopped green olives for a Mediterranean twist. The flavor possibilities are endless!

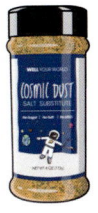

Try our delicious Cosmic Dust in this dish!

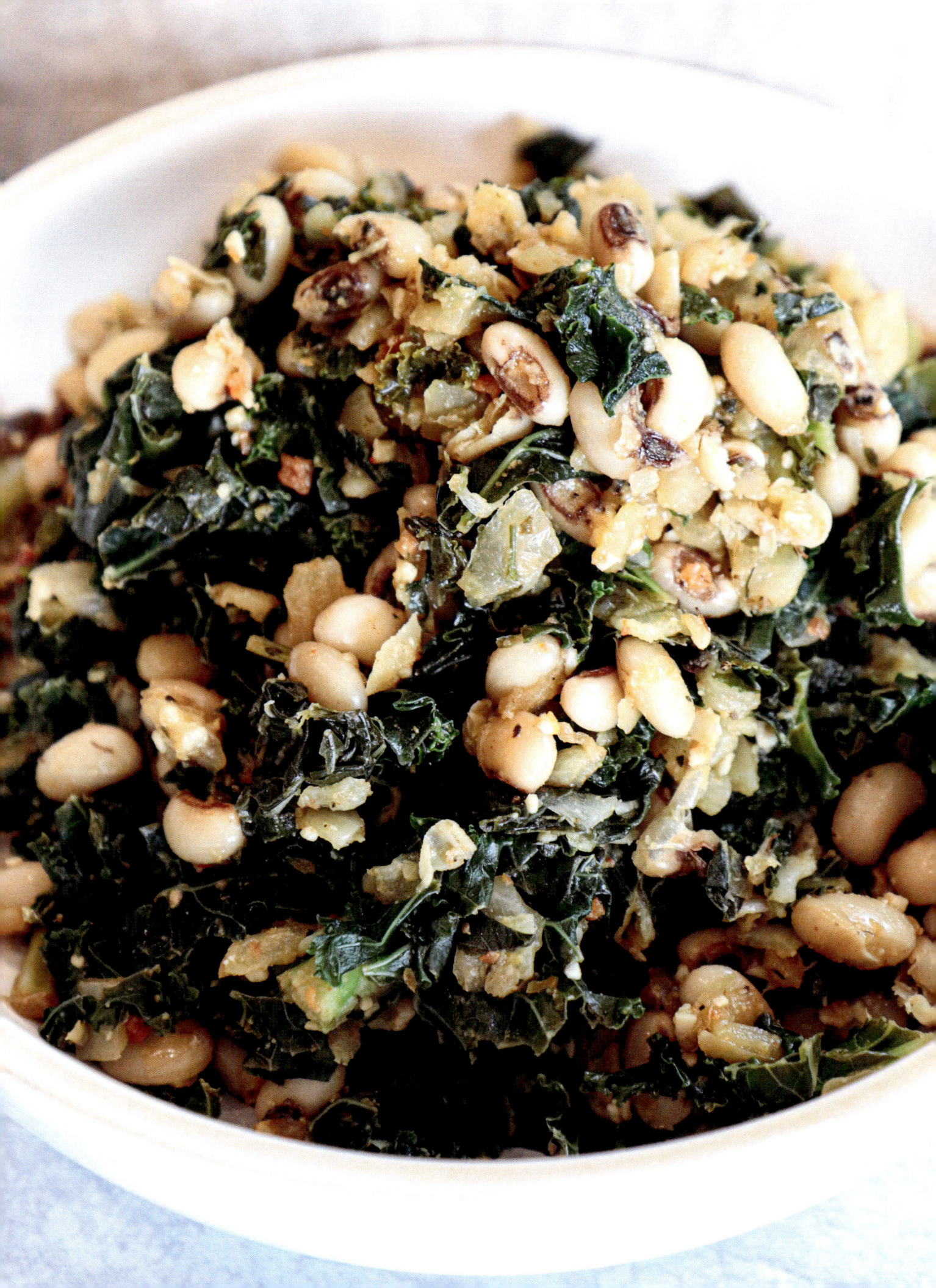

# SPEEDY BLACK-EYED PEAS & GREENS

This perfect pairing of hearty black-eyed peas and nutrient-rich greens creates a satisfying meal in just minutes! Traditional Southern flavors come together in this quick recipe that's both nourishing and delicious.

## INGREDIENTS

- 1   15 oz. can no-salt black eyed peas, drained and rinsed
- 1   10-12 oz. bag frozen chopped onion
- 2-3   teaspoons minced garlic
- 1-2   tablespoons no-salt seasoning
- 2   big handfuls of fresh greens like kale
- 1/2   lemon, juiced

## METHOD

Add the black eyed peas, onion, and garlic to a large saucepan and sauté over medium-high heat for 5-7 minutes until tender, adding veggie broth as needed to keep from sticking.

Add your favorite no-salt seasoning such as Well Your World Cosmic Dust, Italian, or Fiesta and continue to sauté for another minute.

Add the greens and stir continuously until they begin to wilt and integrate with the beans, about 1-2 minutes.

Squeeze fresh lemon juice over the top just before serving. Enjoy!

Note: For even more convenience, try this with frozen greens like kale, spinach, or collards. No chopping required and they cook in the same amount of time!

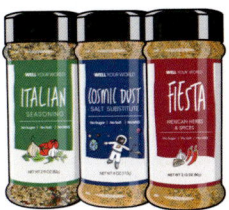

Try our delicious no-salt seasonings in this dish!

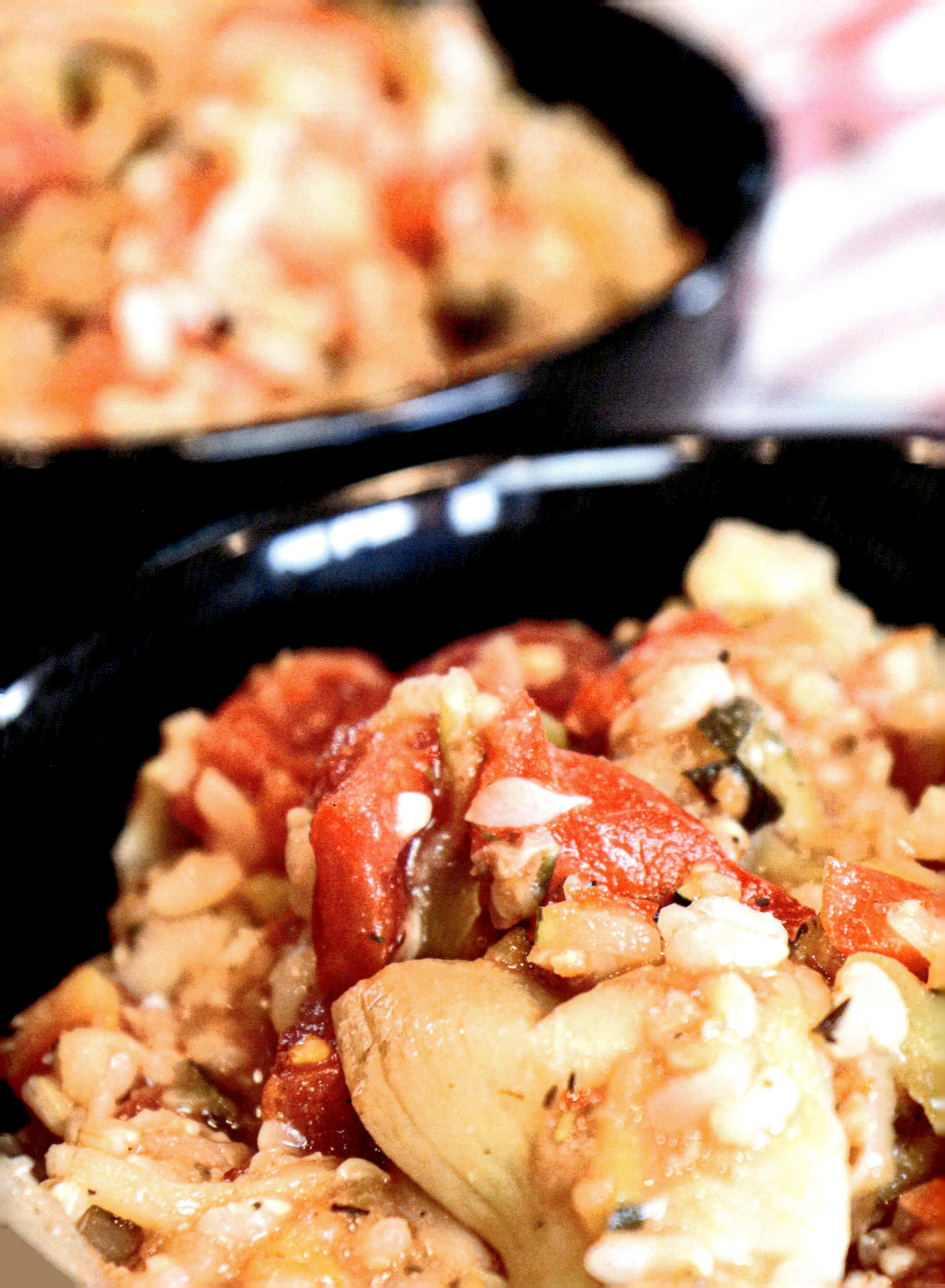

# STOVETOP WOWATOUILLE

This speedy take on classic ratatouille will truly 'wow' your taste buds! Vibrant summer vegetables blend harmoniously with hearty brown rice and zucchini noodles for a satisfying one-pot meal that comes together in minutes.

## INGREDIENTS

- 1 10-12 oz. bag frozen brown rice
- 1 10-12 oz. bag frozen peppers and onions
- 1 10-12 oz. bag frozen (or 1 can) artichoke hearts
- 2 15 oz. cans diced tomatoes
- 1 tablespoon Italian seasoning
- 2 tablespoons nutritional yeast
- 2-3 teaspoons minced garlic
- 1 teaspoon dried basil
- 1 teaspoon crushed red pepper (optional)
- 1 teaspoon date powder
- 1/2 teaspoon dried ground thyme
- 2 10-12 oz. bags frozen "zoodles" (zucchini noodles)

## METHOD

Add everything except the zoodles to a medium dutch oven over high heat. Bring to a boil while stirring occasionally, reduce the heat, and simmer for a few minutes.

Then add the zoodles since they are more fragile than the other ingredients. Stir to bring it all together, simmer to cook through for a minute or two, and enjoy!

Note: No zoodles? Use a spiralizer on fresh zucchini or substitute diced zucchini instead. For a heartier meal, add a can of drained white beans for extra protein and starch.

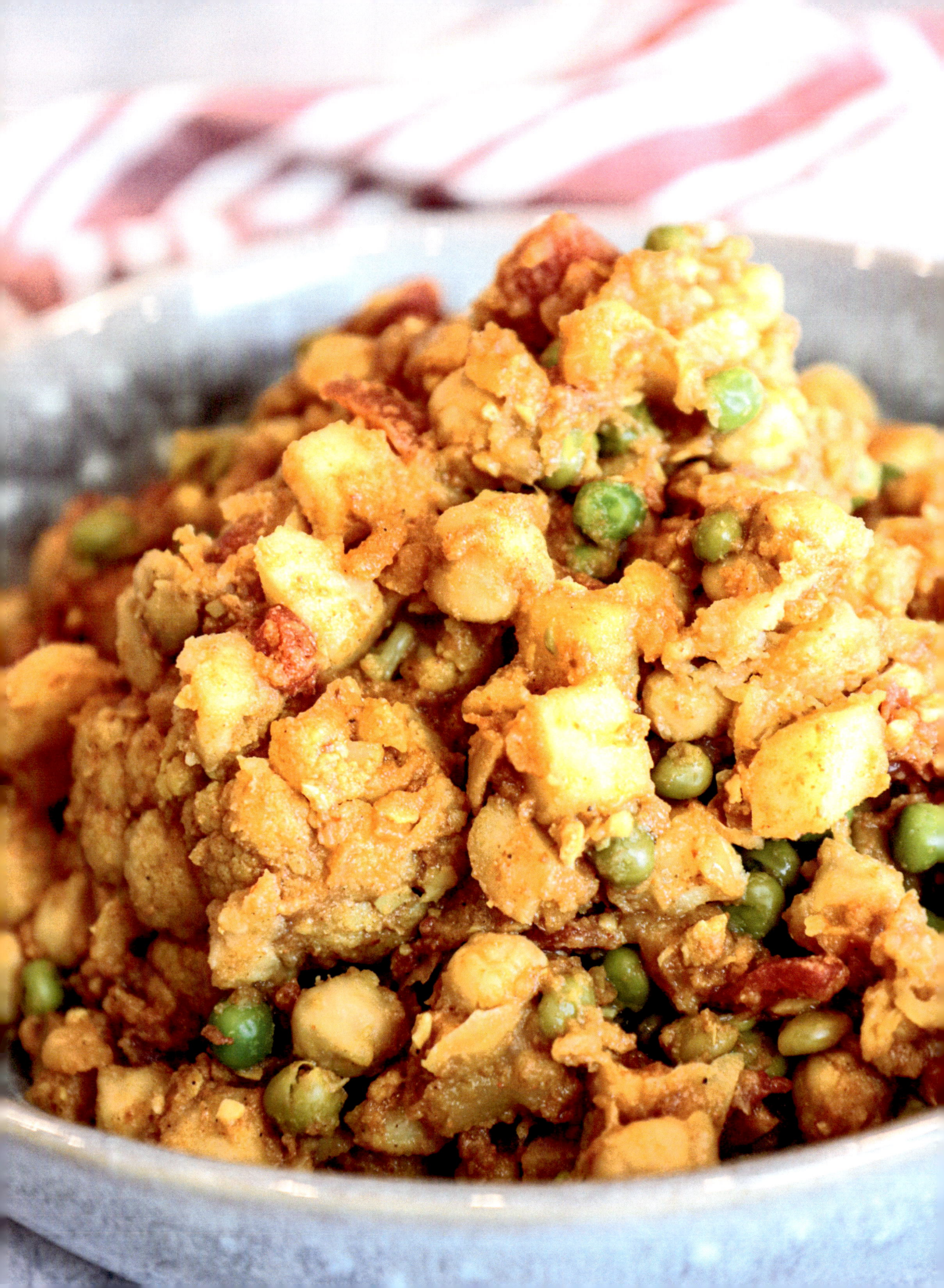

# CURRIED POTATO STEW

This hearty curry-spiced stew combines tender potatoes and chickpeas for a comforting, nutritious meal ready in minutes. Perfect for busy weeknights when you want a satisfying meal without the fuss.

## INGREDIENTS

- 2    15 oz. cans diced tomatoes
- 2    15 oz. cans chickpeas, rinsed and drained
- 1    10-12 oz. bag frozen cauliflower florets
- 1/2  16 oz. bag frozen peas
- 1/2  10-12 oz. bag frozen yellow onion
- 2-3  tablespoons curry powder
- 1    tablespoon minced garlic
- 1    tablespoon nutritional yeast
- 1    teaspoon chili powder
- 1/2  1 lb. bag frozen cubed potatoes

  fresh chopped cilantro, to serve

## METHOD

Add everything except the potatoes to a large pot and bring to a boil. Reduce the heat and simmer for a minute, then toss in the potatoes and let simmer for a couple more minutes, stirring occasionally until potatoes are just tender.

Top with fresh chopped cilantro and enjoy!

---

Note: For a creamier stew, mash some of the chickpeas before adding to the pot. Try adding a handful of spinach in the last minute of cooking for extra nutrition and color. Delicious served over brown rice or with whole grain flatbread.

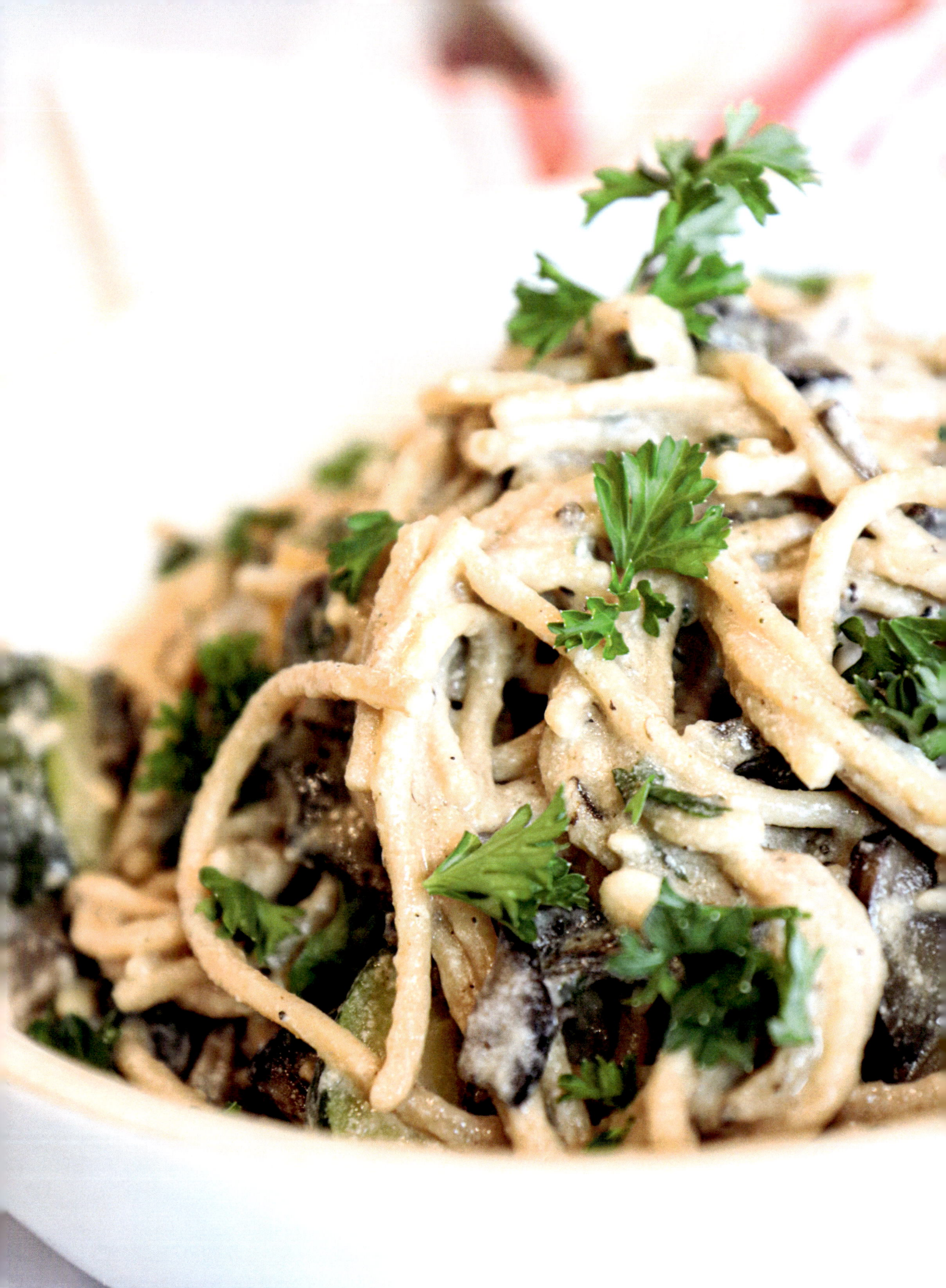

# PASTA CARBONARA

This carbonara delivers all the creamy, smoky flavor of the Italian classic. Savory mushrooms and tender pasta combine with a rich, silky sauce for a satisfying meal that comes together quickly.

## INGREDIENTS

- 1/2 lb. whole wheat spaghetti
- 1 10-12 oz. bag frozen chopped zucchini

### Sauce
- 1/2 lb. fresh or frozen chopped mushrooms
- 1/2 teaspoon liquid smoke
- 2 cups soy milk
- 1/4 cup nutritional yeast
- 1/4 cup sun-dried tomatoes, chopped
- 1 tablespoon chickpea flour
- 1 tablespoon capers or lemon juice
- 2-3 teaspoons minced garlic
- 2 teaspoons onion powder
- 1/4 teaspoon black pepper
- 1/4 teaspoon ground nutmeg
- 1/4 teaspoon dried thyme
- 1/2 cup fresh chopped parsley

- 2 tablespoons pine nuts (optional)

## METHOD

Cook the pasta according to package directions in an extra large pot of water. During the last two minutes of cooking, add the frozen zucchini to cook with the boiling pasta. Then drain and set aside.

While the pasta is cooking, prepare the sauce. Add the mushrooms to a saucepan and sauté over medium-high heat for a couple minutes, adding a splash of water or veggie broth as needed to keep from sticking. Add the liquid smoke and continue to sauté until the mushrooms shrink. Then whisk in the soy milk and the rest of the ingredients except the parsley and pine nuts.

Bring the sauce up to a boil, reduce heat, and simmer for a few minutes. Then mix in the parsley.

Finally, toss the pasta and zucchini in with the sauce, stir to combine, top with pine nuts, and enjoy!

Note: We love the bags of plain sun-dried tomatoes for this recipe. Trader Joe's has a great option, but many brands work well. For a more traditional carbonara texture, reduce or omit the chickpea flour for a thinner sauce.

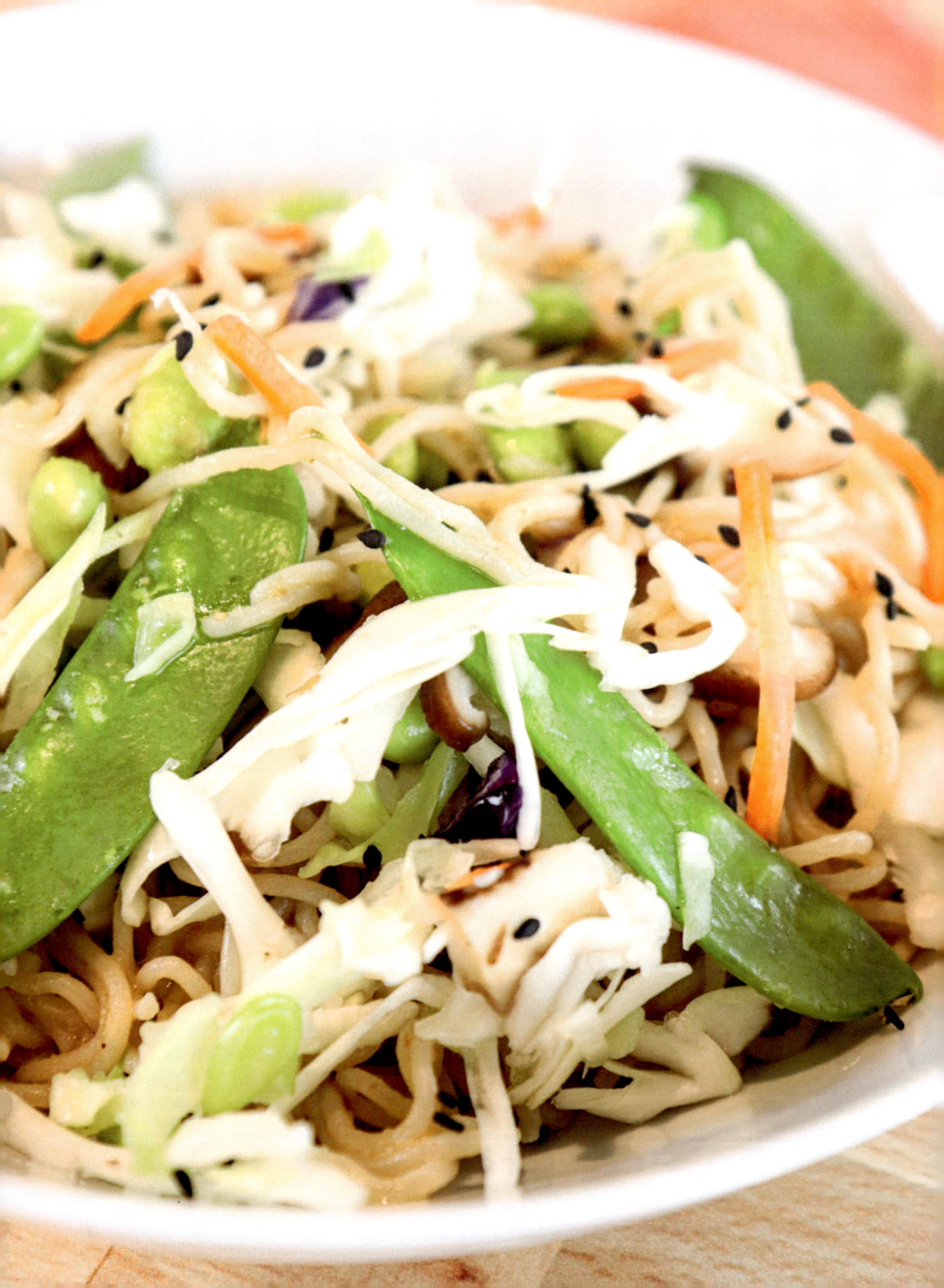

# TERIYAKI STIR FRY

This vibrant stir fry combines crisp vegetables and tender noodles in a homemade teriyaki sauce. Ready in just minutes, it delivers bold flavor and satisfying textures with minimal effort.

## INGREDIENTS

### Teriyaki Sauce
- 1/4 cup frozen pineapple, thawed
- 5 tablespoons water
- 3 tablespoons rice vinegar
- 1 tablespoon tamari (optional)
- 1 teaspoon sriracha
- 6 deglet dates
- 2 garlic cloves
- 1 green onion
- 1/2" nub fresh ginger

### Stir Fry
- 1-2 blocks ramen noodles
- 1 large handful fresh snow peas
- 1/2 14-16 oz. bag frozen onion and bell pepper mix
- 1/2 14-16 oz. bag frozen San Fran Blend (green beans, broccoli, onions, mushrooms, and red bell pepper)
- 1/4 14-16 oz. bag frozen peas and carrots mix
- 1/2 8 oz. can water chestnuts, drained

  green onions, to serve
  black sesame seeds, to serve

## METHOD

To prepare the Teriyaki Sauce, add all of the ingredients to a small bullet blender and blend until smooth. Set aside.

Bring a medium-sized pot of water to a boil and add the ramen noodles. Cook according to package directions. During the final 2-3 minutes, add all the frozen and canned vegetables to the same pot, turn the heat to high, and cook until the noodles are tender and vegetables are heated through.

Drain the veggies and noodles, then add them back to the pot along with the Teriyaki Sauce. Cook for another minute or two just to heat everything back up. Top with green onions and sesame seeds and enjoy!

Note: We love the Lotus Foods brand Millet & Brown Rice Ramen noodles for this dish. For extra richness, add a cup of edamame or a block of cubed tofu with the vegetables. This meal makes excellent leftovers for lunch the next day!

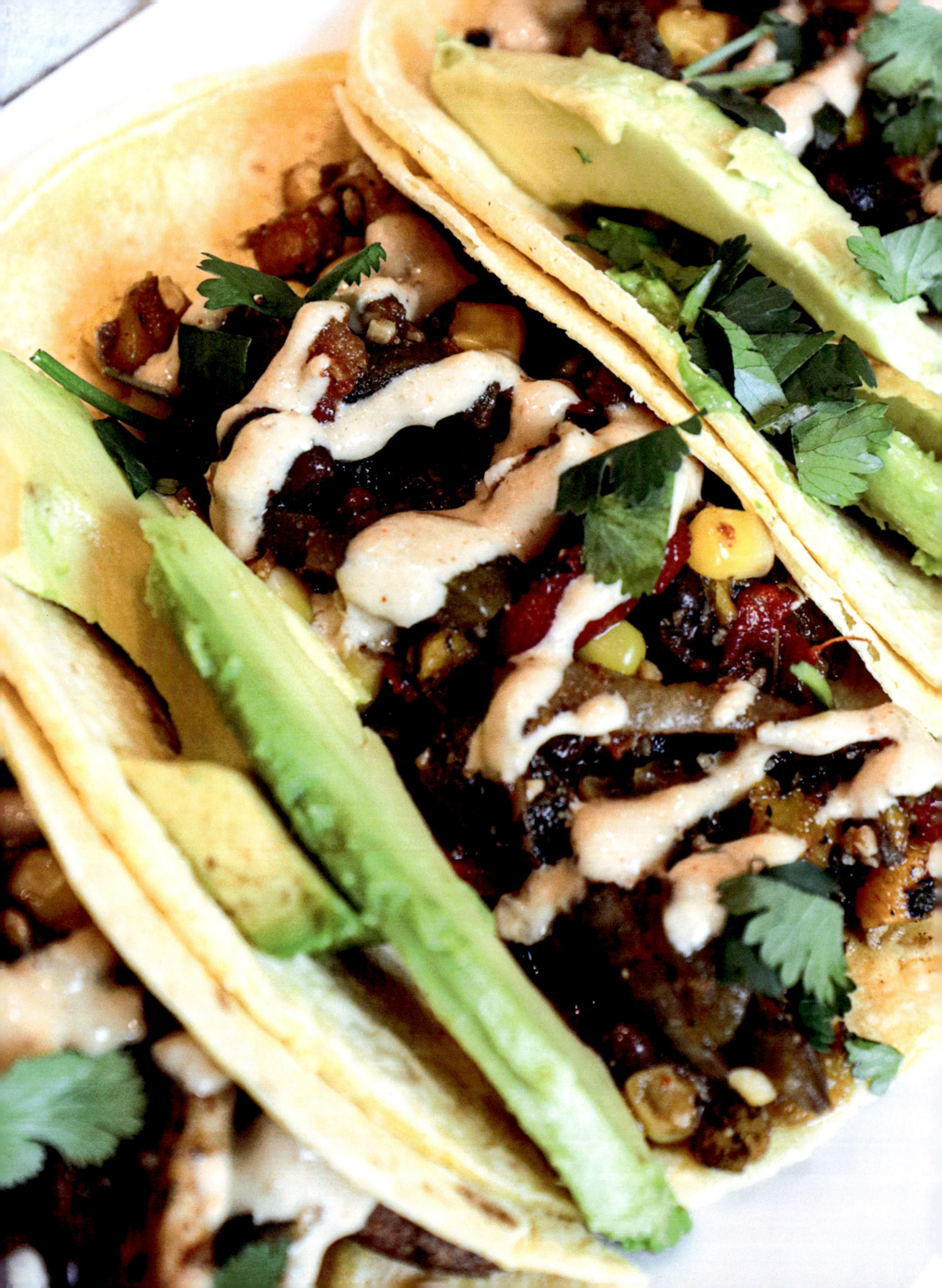

# VEGGIE FAJITAS

These vibrant fajitas combine sautéed peppers, onions, and mushrooms with hearty black beans. Paired with a zesty, creamy tahini sauce, they make a quick and satisfying meal the whole family will love.

## INGREDIENTS

**Veggie Fajitas**

- 1   10-12 oz. bag frozen bell pepper and onion strips
- 1   portobello mushroom, sliced
- 1   15 oz. can black beans, drained and rinsed
- 1/2   cup frozen char roasted corn
- 2   teaspoons dried oregano
- 1   teaspoon ground cumin
- 1   teaspoon paprika
- 1/2   teaspoon chili powder

**I-Need-A Fajita Sauce**

- 1/4   cup tahini
- 2   teaspoons nutritional yeast
- 1   teaspoon garlic powder
- 1   teaspoon onion powder
- 1/2   teaspoon paprika
- 1/2   teaspoon cayenne pepper
- 2   deglet dates
- 1/2   lime, juiced
- water to reach desired consistency

**Serve With**

- corn tortillas
- I-Need-A Fajita Sauce
- pico de gallo
- broccoli slaw or coleslaw mix
- fresh cilantro, chopped
- avocado

## METHOD

To prepare the Veggie Fajitas, add all the ingredients to a large skillet and sauté over medium-high heat, adding a little water or veggie broth as needed to keep from sticking. Cook until vegetables are tender, about 5 minutes. Remove from heat.

To prepare the I-Need-A Fajita Sauce, add all the ingredients to a high-speed blender and blend until smooth. Start with 2 tablespoons of water and add more as needed until you reach your desired consistency.

To make the perfect taco, stack some fajita veggies on a corn tortilla with a drizzle of I-Need-A Fajita Sauce, pico, slaw, avocado, and chopped cilantro!

**Note: For even quicker preparation, use 1-2 tablespoons of our Fiesta, Chile Lime, Red Chile, or Green Chile seasoning instead of measuring individual spices!**

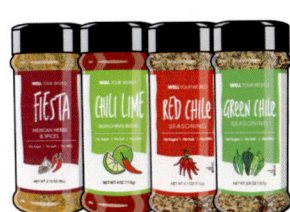

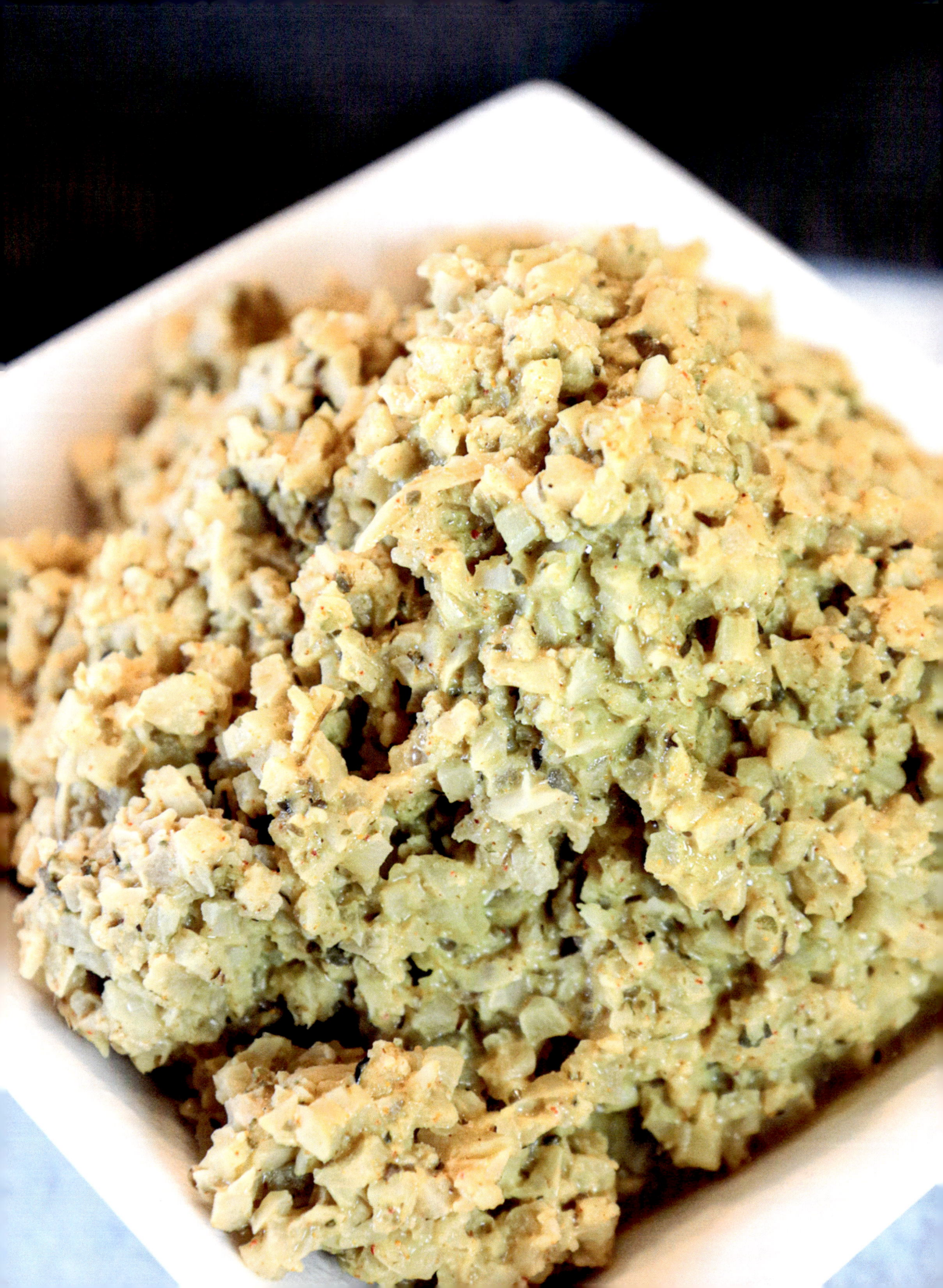

# REEBS' RICED CAULIFLOWER

This savory riced cauliflower dish delivers cheesy flavor without the dairy. Ready in minutes, it makes a versatile side that works perfectly on its own or as a base for bowls and salads.

## INGREDIENTS

- 1      10-12 oz. bag frozen riced cauliflower
- 3/4    cup soy milk
- 1/4    cup nutritional yeast
- 2      teaspoons dried oregano
- 1      teaspoon onion powder
- 1/2-1  teaspoon chili powder
- 1/2    teaspoon ground cumin

## METHOD

Add all of the ingredients to a small saucepan, stir well to combine, and simmer over medium heat for 4-6 minutes or until heated through. Enjoy!

You can also make a half-sized version in a microwave-safe bowl by microwaving on high for 2-3 minutes, stirring halfway through.

For a more filling meal, sub the cauliflower for a bag of frozen rice or use a combination of both.

Note: For even faster preparation, try using our Fiesta Blend! Just use 1-2 tablespoons instead of measuring all the individual spices. This also works beautifully as a stuffing for bell peppers or as a base layer in burritos.

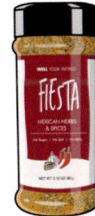

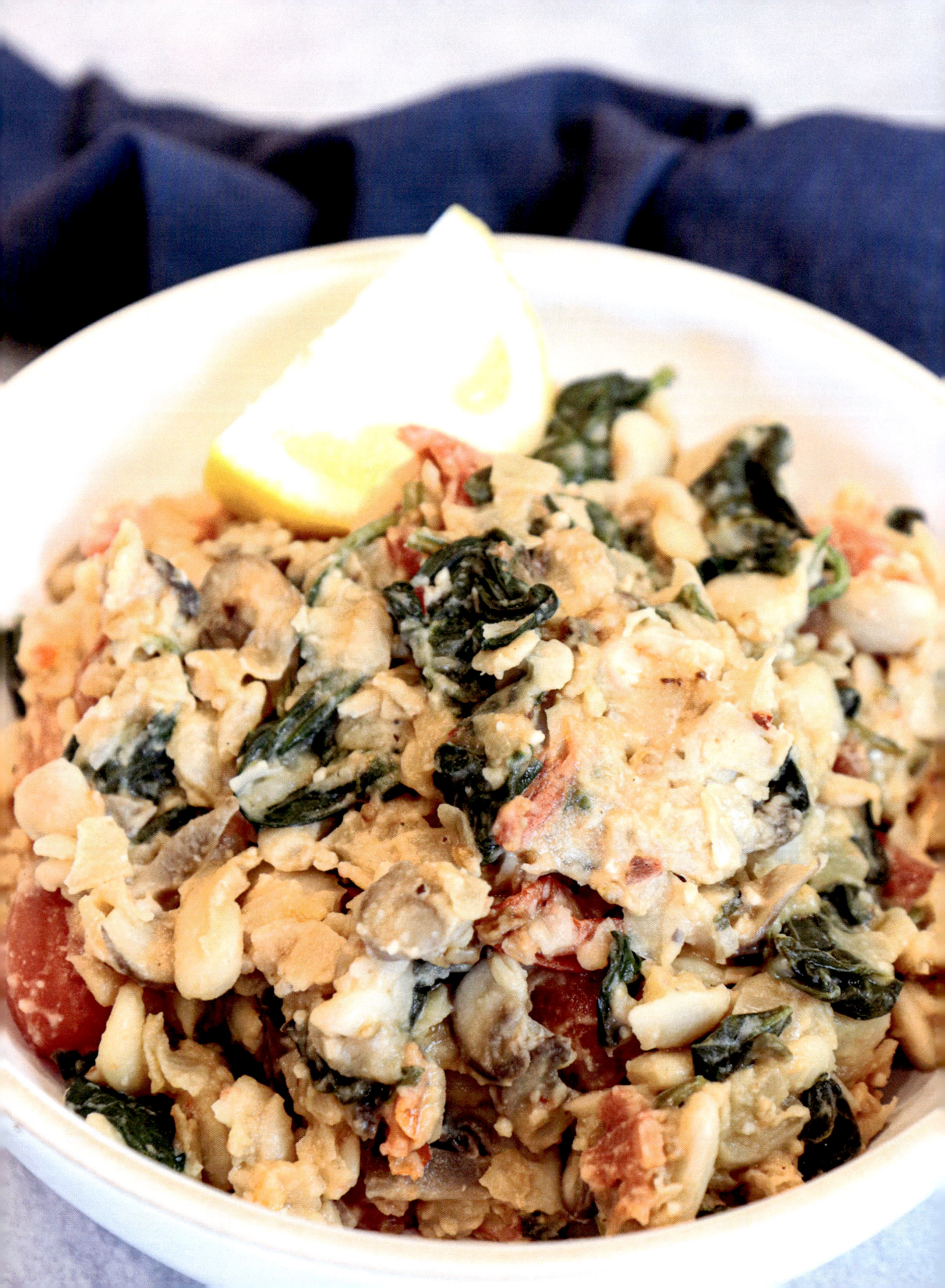

# CREAMY BUTTER BEANS

These velvety butter beans are enveloped in a rich, homemade hummus sauce with savory mushrooms and sweet cherry tomatoes. This hearty dish comes together quickly and delivers restaurant-quality flavor in minutes.

## INGREDIENTS

### Hummus
- 1 15 oz. can chickpeas
- 1/2 cup aquafaba (bean liquid)
- 1 lemon, juiced
- 4 garlic cloves
- 1 teaspoon smoked paprika
- 1/2 teaspoon ground cumin
- 1/2 teaspoon liquid smoke
- 2 tablespoons tahini (optional)

### Butter Beans
- 1 10-12 oz. bag frozen chopped onion
- 6-8 mushrooms, chopped (optional)
- 1/2 pint cherry tomatoes
- 3 garlic cloves, minced
- 2 teaspoons date powder
- 1/2 teaspoon liquid smoke (optional)
- 1/4 teaspoon crushed red pepper (optional)
- 1/4 teaspoon black pepper
- 3 tablespoons Hummus
- 2 handfuls baby spinach
- 1 15 oz. can butter beans, drained and rinsed
- 1 lemon, juiced to serve

## METHOD

To prepare the hummus, add all of the ingredients to a high-speed blender and blend until smooth, using the plunger continuously to push the mixture down as it blends. Set aside.

To prepare the dish, add the onion, mushrooms, and tomatoes to a pan and sauté over medium-high heat for a few minutes, adding a little water or veggie broth as needed to keep from sticking.

Then add the garlic, date powder, liquid smoke, crushed red pepper, and black pepper and continue to sauté for a couple minutes. Next, stir in the Hummus and continue to sauté for another minute.

Finally, add the spinach and butter beans. Stir gently until the spinach has wilted, then remove from heat. If you left the tomatoes whole, you can use a potato masher to break them apart for a chunkier sauce texture.

Stir in the lemon juice and enjoy!

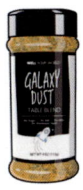

*Try our delicious Galaxy Dust Seasoning Blend in this dish!*

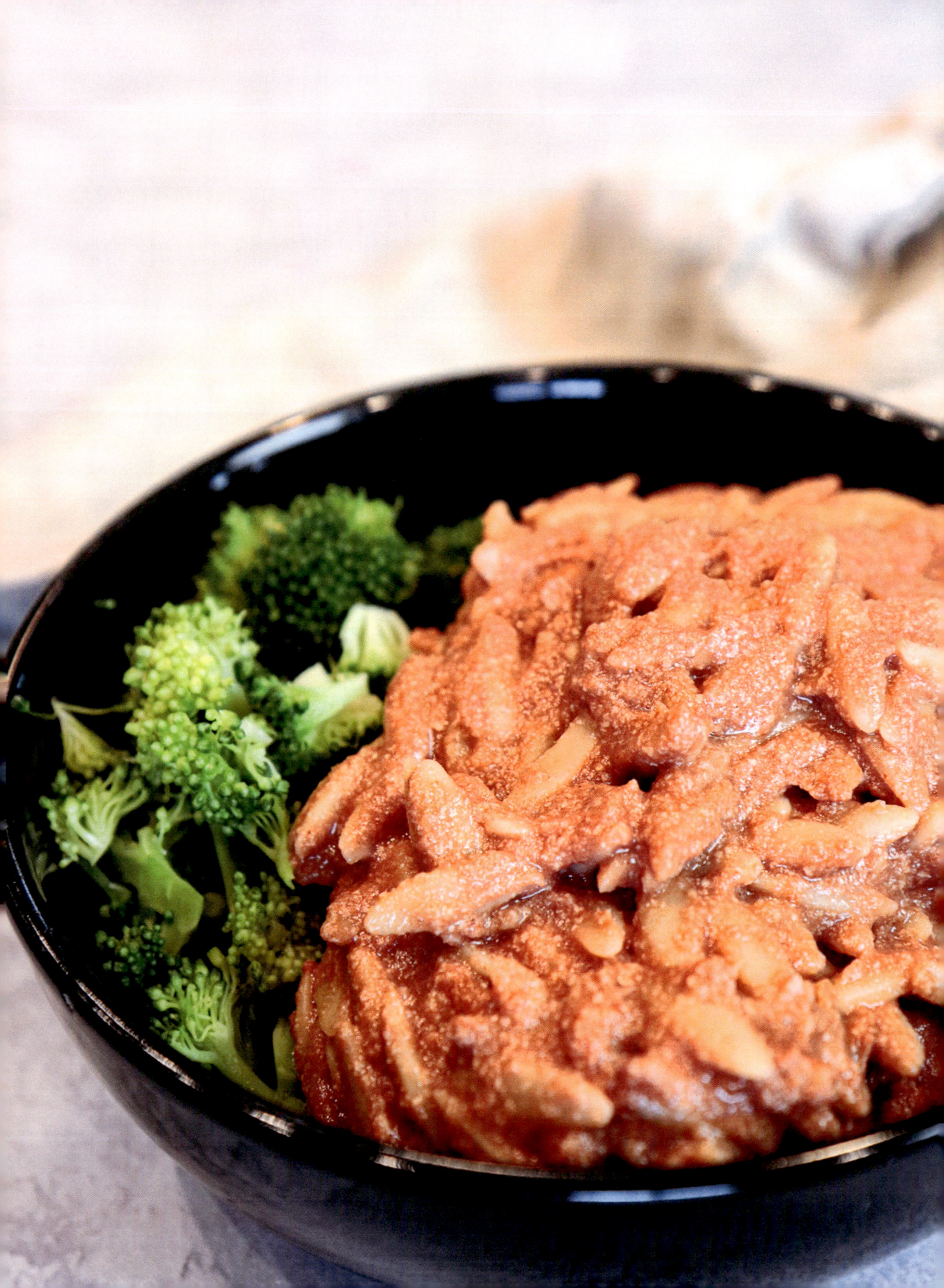

# SPAGHETTI ORZ-O'S

This nostalgic spin on a childhood favorite delivers all the comfort of the classic canned meal but with wholesome ingredients. Tender orzo pasta in a rich, savory tomato sauce makes for a quick, satisfying dish that both kids and adults will love.

## INGREDIENTS

- 5 oz. whole wheat orzo
- 1 15 oz. can tomato sauce
- 1/4 cup nutritional yeast
- 2 tablespoons soy milk
- 1 tablespoon date powder
- 1/2 teaspoon onion powder
- 1/2 teaspoon garlic powder
- 1/2 teaspoon paprika

## METHOD

Prepare the pasta according to the package directions and set aside.

While the pasta is cooking, add all remaining ingredients to a separate saucepan. Whisk together thoroughly and slowly bring to a gentle boil over medium heat, stirring occasionally. Use a lid to prevent splattering as the sauce heats.

Add the pasta to the sauce, stir, simmer for a minute, and enjoy!

Note: Optionally, add chopped broccoli or zucchini during the last few minutes of boiling the pasta. They'll cook perfectly alongside the orzo and add color, texture, and nutrients. For extra protein, stir a can of drained and rinsed white beans into the sauce.

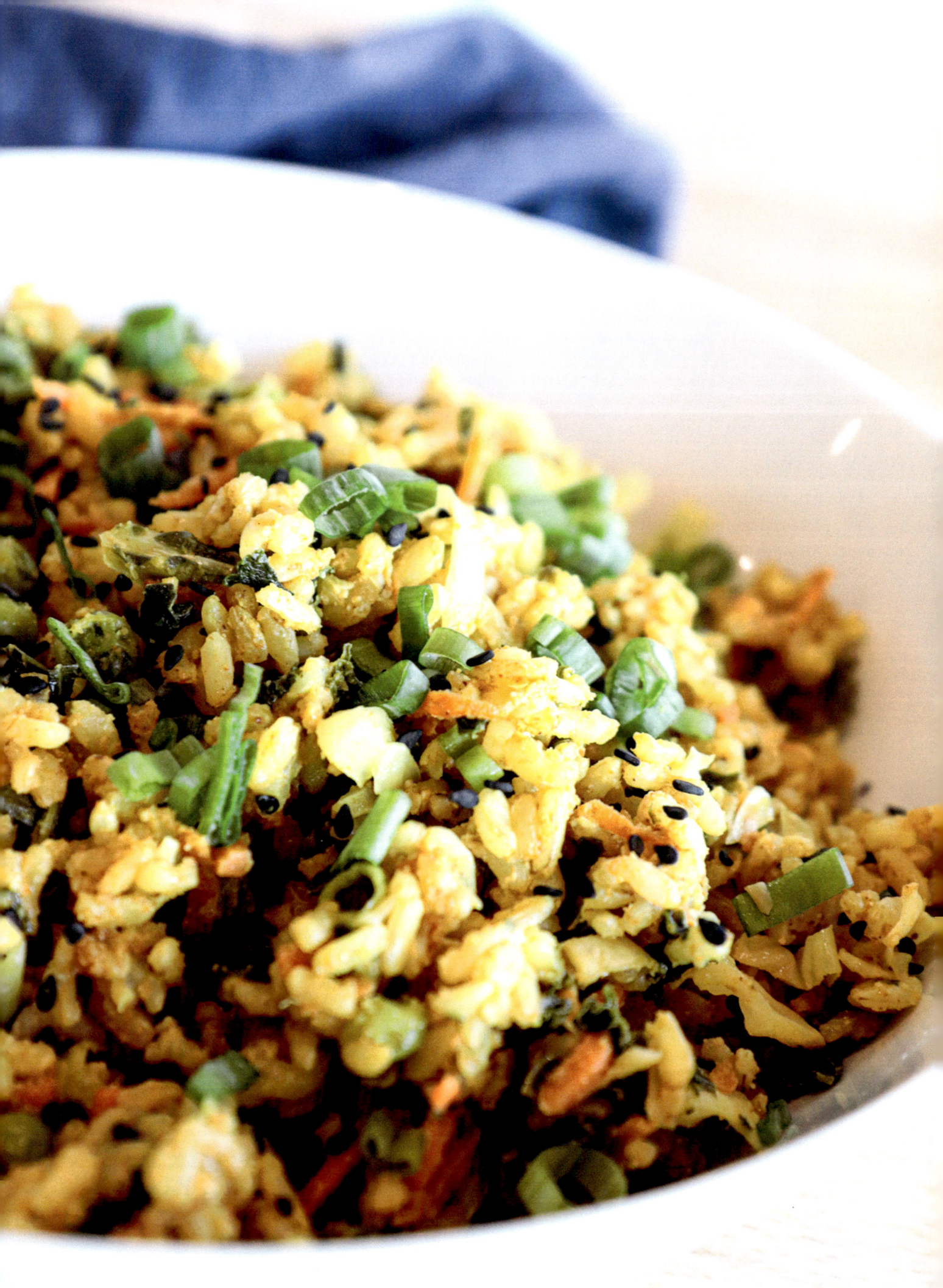

# MICROWAVED FRIED RICE

This clever microwave method turns simple ingredients into a satisfying 'fried' rice in minutes. Perfect for dorm rooms, office lunches, or anytime you need a quick meal without access to a full kitchen—all the flavor with minimal equipment!

## INGREDIENTS

- 1 10-12 oz. bag frozen rice
- 1 handful frozen peas
- 1 handful frozen chopped kale
- 1 handful shredded carrots
- 1 handful coleslaw mix (cabbage)
- 1 tablespoon rice vinegar
- 1 tablespoon peanut butter (optional)
- 1-2 teaspoons tamari (optional)
- 1 teaspoon garlic powder
- 1 teaspoon onion powder
- 1 teaspoon ground ginger
- 1 teaspoon ground cumin
- 1/4 teaspoon ground turmeric

- chopped green onion, to serve
- sesame seeds, to serve

## METHOD

Add all ingredients to a large mixing bowl and toss until well combined. Transfer to a microwave-safe bowl and microwave uncovered for about 5 minutes, stopping halfway to stir for more even cooking.

Once cooked, fluff the rice mixture with a fork to separate the grains and distribute the seasonings. Top with chopped green onions and sesame seeds. Enjoy!

Note: Customize with your favorite add-ins like pineapple, edamame, or diced tofu! For a spicier version, add a teaspoon of sriracha or a pinch of crushed red pepper. This recipe works well with leftover cooked rice too.

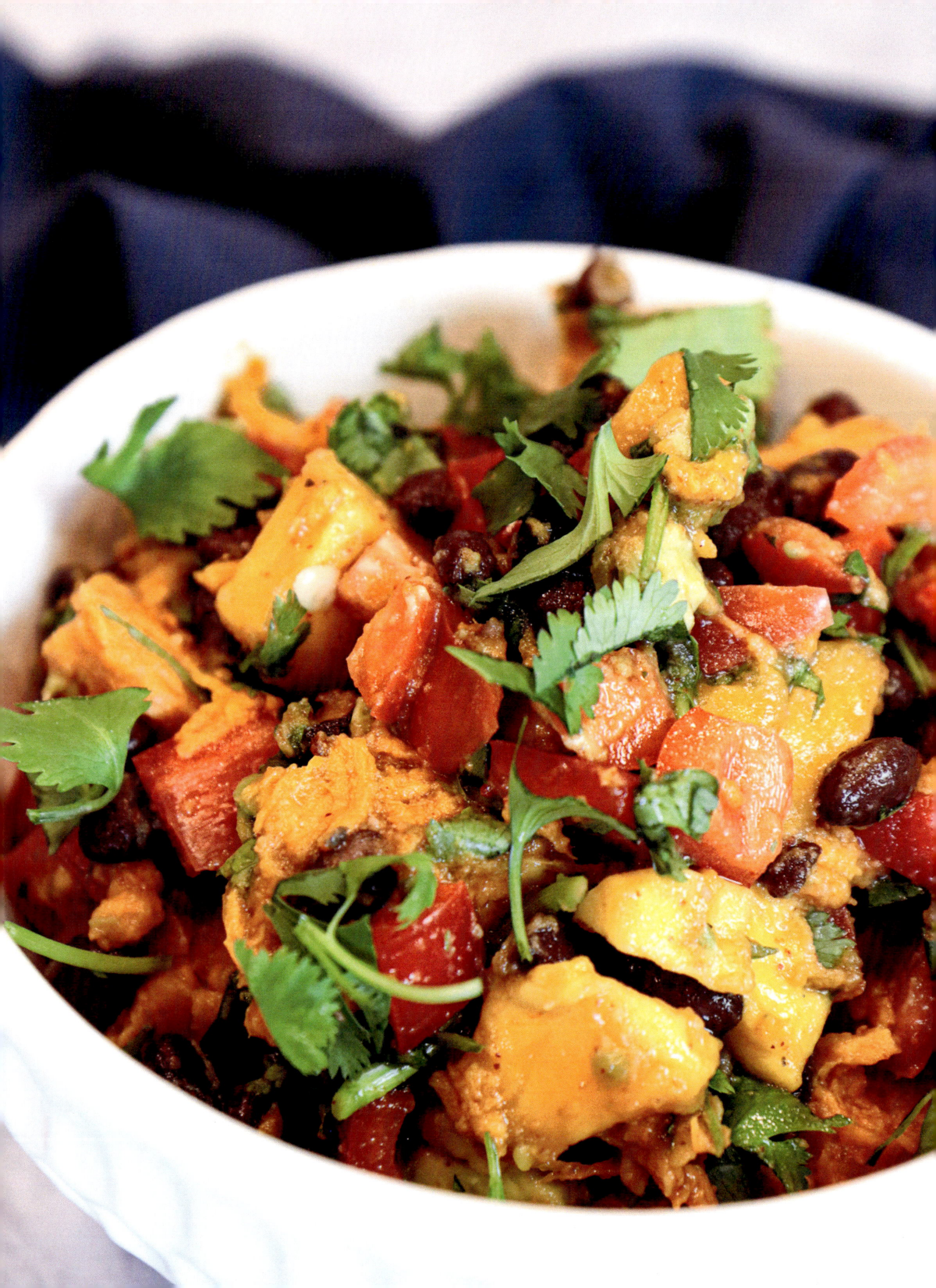

# SWEET POTATO BLACK BEAN BOWL

This vibrant bowl combines hearty sweet potatoes with protein-rich black beans, sweet mango, and creamy avocado. Finished with a tangy balsamic drizzle, it delivers a perfect balance of flavors and textures in just minutes—no cooking required!

## INGREDIENTS

- 1 large sweet potato, cooked, peeled, cubed, and cooled
- 2 cups frozen mango, thawed and chopped
- 1 red bell pepper, diced
- 1 15 oz. can black beans, drained and rinsed
- 1 avocado, diced
- 1 jalapeño, seeded and diced (optional)
- 1 handful cilantro, chopped
- 1 lime, juiced
- 1-2 teaspoons WYW Chili Lime Seasoning (optional)
- 1-2 teaspoons WYW Calypso Seasoning (optional)
- balsamic vinegar, to taste

## METHOD

If you don't have pre-cooked sweet potatoes, boil cubed sweet potato for about 10 minutes or until tender. Drain and let cool before using.

Add all the ingredients except the balsamic vinegar to a bowl and toss gently to combine. Drizzle with balsamic vinegar and give it one final toss to evenly coat all ingredients.

Enjoy this bowl on its own, wrapped in a tortilla, over a bed of fresh greens, or alongside your favorite whole grains for a well-rounded meal!

Note: We often use meal-prepped sweet potatoes from the fridge for super-quick assembly. The WYW Calypso Caribbean Seasoning Blend really makes this dish pop with tropical flavors!

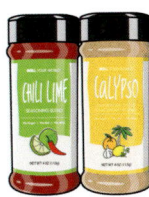

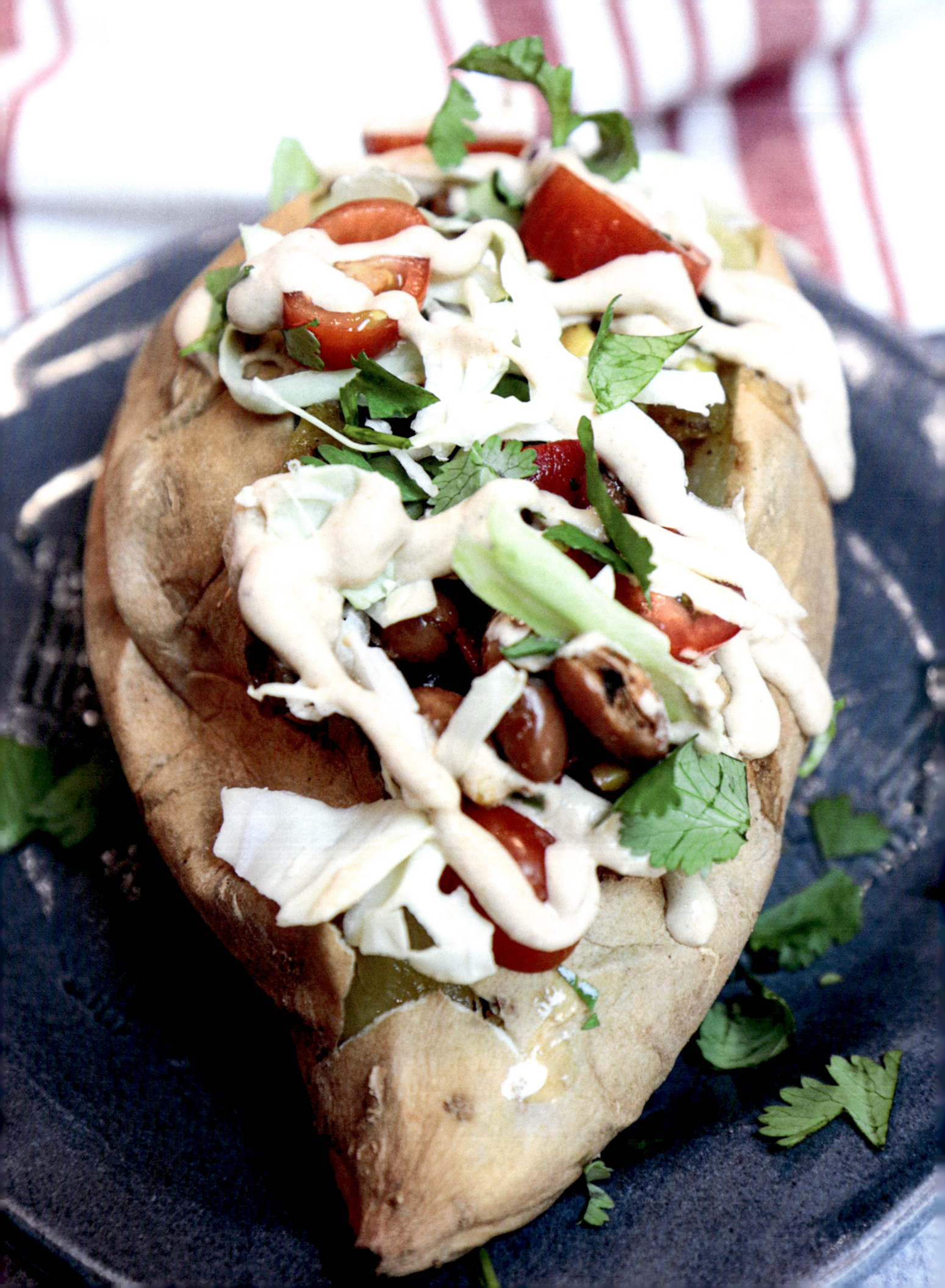

# STUFFED SWEET POTATOES

These satisfying stuffed sweet potatoes combine hearty, starchy goodness with a flavorful bean and veggie filling. Topped with a creamy chipotle aioli, they deliver a perfect balance of sweet, smoky, and savory in every bite.

## INGREDIENTS

### Chipotle Aioli
- 1/2 cup cashews
- 1/2 cup soy milk + tablespoon as needed
- 1 1/2 teaspoons chipotle powder
- 2 garlic cloves
- 2 deglet dates
- 1 lime, juiced

### Stuffed Sweet Potatoes
- 4 sweet potatoes
- 1 15 oz. can pinto beans, drained and rinsed
- 1 12-14 oz. bag frozen char roasted onion & bell peppers
- 1/2 cup frozen char roasted corn
- 1 teaspoon ground cumin
- 1 teaspoon smoked paprika
- 1 teaspoon dried oregano
- 1/2 teaspoon crushed red pepper or black pepper, to taste

### Serve With
- cherry tomatoes, chopped
- fresh cilantro, chopped
- coleslaw mix
- Chipotle Aioli

## METHOD

To prepare the Chipotle Aioli, add all of the ingredients to a high-speed blender and blend until smooth. Add an additional splash of soy milk as needed to reach your desired consistency. Set aside.

Use a fork to poke several holes in the sweet potatoes to allow steam to escape. Microwave two potatoes at a time for 5-7 minutes, turning halfway through cooking, until they yield easily when squeezed (careful, they'll be hot!).

Meanwhile, prepare the filling by adding all remaining ingredients to a saucepan. Sauté over medium-high heat, adding a little water or veggie broth as needed to keep from sticking. Cook until everything is heated through and vegetables are tender, about 5 minutes.

Make a lengthwise cut down the sweet potatoes and spoon in some filling. Top with cherry tomatoes, cilantro, coleslaw mix, and Chipotle Aioli. Enjoy!

Note: To batch cook sweet potatoes for the week, bake them in the oven at 400°F for an hour or until tender. They'll keep in the fridge for up to a week for quick meals.

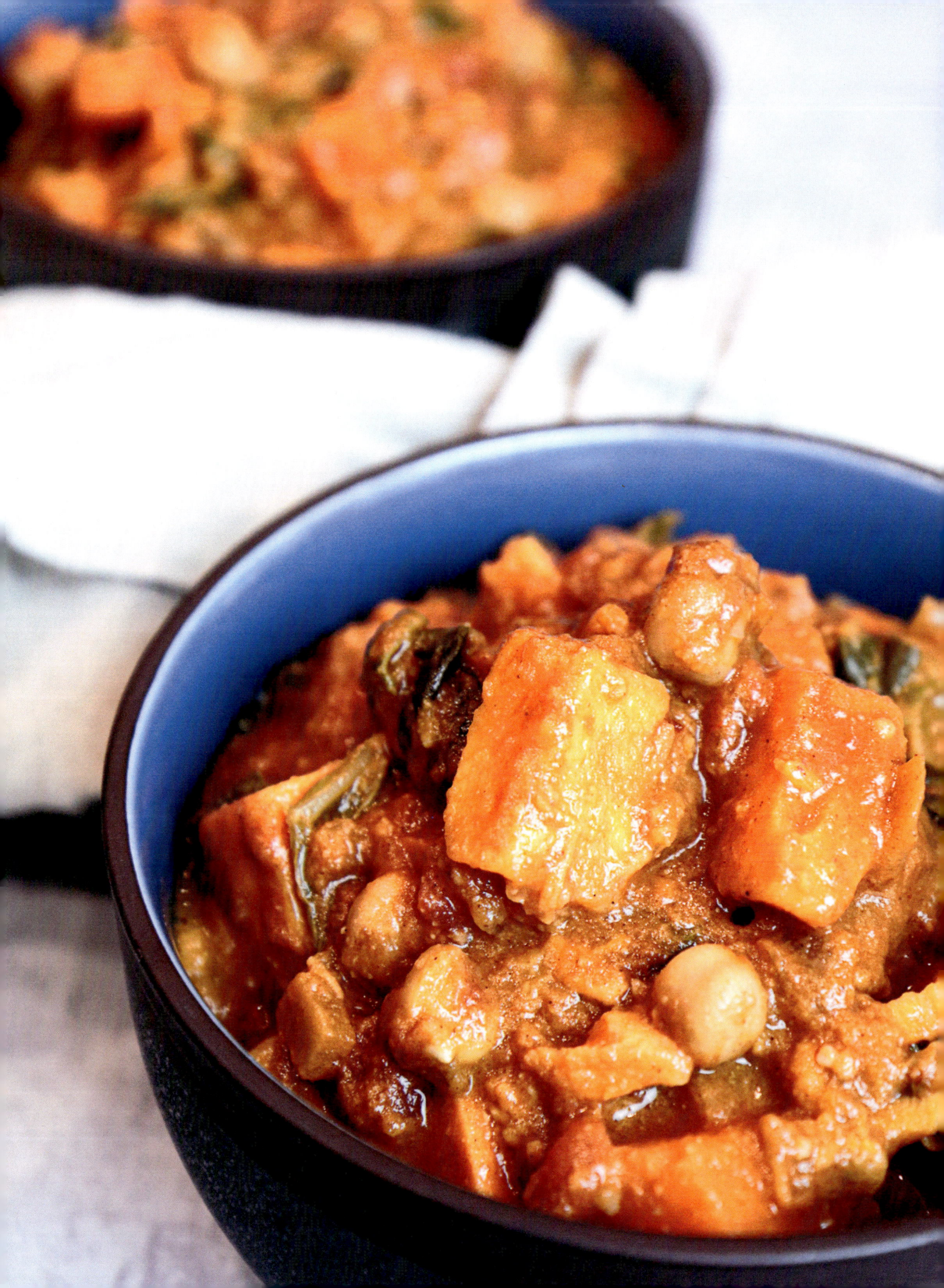

# AFRICAN PEANUT STEW

This hearty stew combines creamy peanut butter with nutrient-rich vegetables and warming spices. Featuring butternut squash, sweet potatoes, and chickpeas in a flavorful tomato base, it's a quick one-pot meal that tastes like it's been simmering all day.

## INGREDIENTS

- 2 10-12 oz. bags frozen cubed sweet potato or butternut squash
- 1 10-12 oz. bag frozen chopped onion
- 1 15 oz. can diced tomatoes
- 1 15 oz. can tomato sauce
- 1 15 oz. can chickpeas, drained and rinsed
- 1 bunch collard greens or kale, destemmed and chopped
- 4 cups veggie broth
- 2 tablespoons peanut butter
- 1 tablespoon minced garlic
- 2 teaspoons ground cumin
- 1 teaspoon dried ground ginger
- 1 teaspoon ground cinnamon
- 1 teaspoon ground coriander
- 1/4 teaspoon crushed red pepper (optional)

## METHOD

Add all of the ingredients to a large pot and bring to a boil, stirring occasionally to prevent sticking. Reduce the heat and let simmer for 5-30 minutes - the longer it cooks, the more the flavors will develop, but it's delicious either way!

Serve and enjoy!

---

Note: For an even quicker version, use frozen chopped collard greens or kale instead of fresh. This stew freezes beautifully for meal prep and tastes even better the next day. Serve over brown rice or quinoa to make it even more filling!

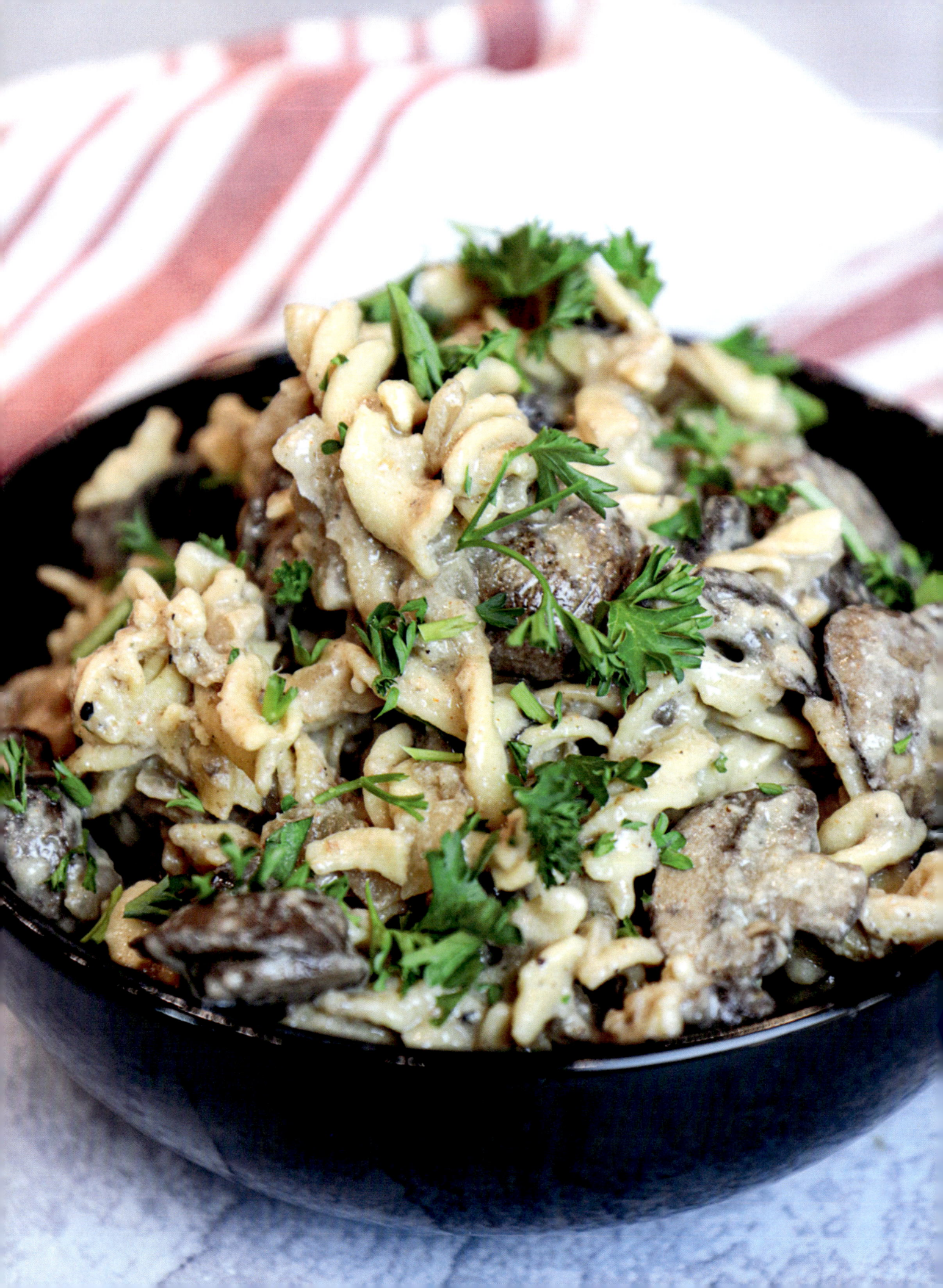

# MUSHROOM STROGANOFF

This creamy, savory stroganoff transforms earthy mushrooms into a restaurant-quality meal in minutes. The velvety sauce coats every bite with rich flavor, making this quick version a weeknight dinner you'll return to again and again.

## INGREDIENTS

- 8 oz. whole wheat or bean pasta
- 1 10-12 oz. bag frozen chopped onion
- 1 16 oz. package fresh sliced mushrooms
- 1 tablespoon minced garlic
- 2 tablespoons nutritional yeast
- 1 tablespoon white wine vinegar or lemon juice
- 1 tablespoon dijon mustard
- 1-2 teaspoons tamari (optional)
- 1/2 teaspoon dried thyme
- 1/2 teaspoon black pepper
- 1/2 teaspoon smoked paprika
- 1 cup soy milk
- 1 cup veggie broth
- 2 tablespoons whole wheat flour
- 1 handful fresh parsley, chopped

## METHOD

Prepare the pasta according to the package directions and set aside.

Add the onions, mushrooms, and garlic to a saucepan and sauté over medium-high heat for 3-5 minutes, adding a little water or veggie broth as needed to keep from sticking. Cook until mushrooms release their moisture and begin to brown.

Next, add the nutritional yeast through the paprika and continue to sauté for a couple more minutes.

Then add the soy milk and veggie broth, and stir well. Gradually sprinkle and whisk in the flour to prevent lumps. Simmer for 2-3 minutes, stirring frequently until the sauce thickens.

Add the pasta to the saucepan and stir to combine. Serve topped with fresh chopped parsley along with more black pepper as desired. Enjoy!

Note: This stroganoff sauce works over any starch—sweet potatoes, rice, or quinoa. For a shortcut, use our Mushroom Gravy Mix as the sauce base: just prepare per package directions and add to the sautéed mushrooms and onions.

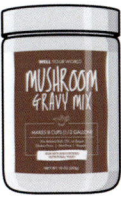

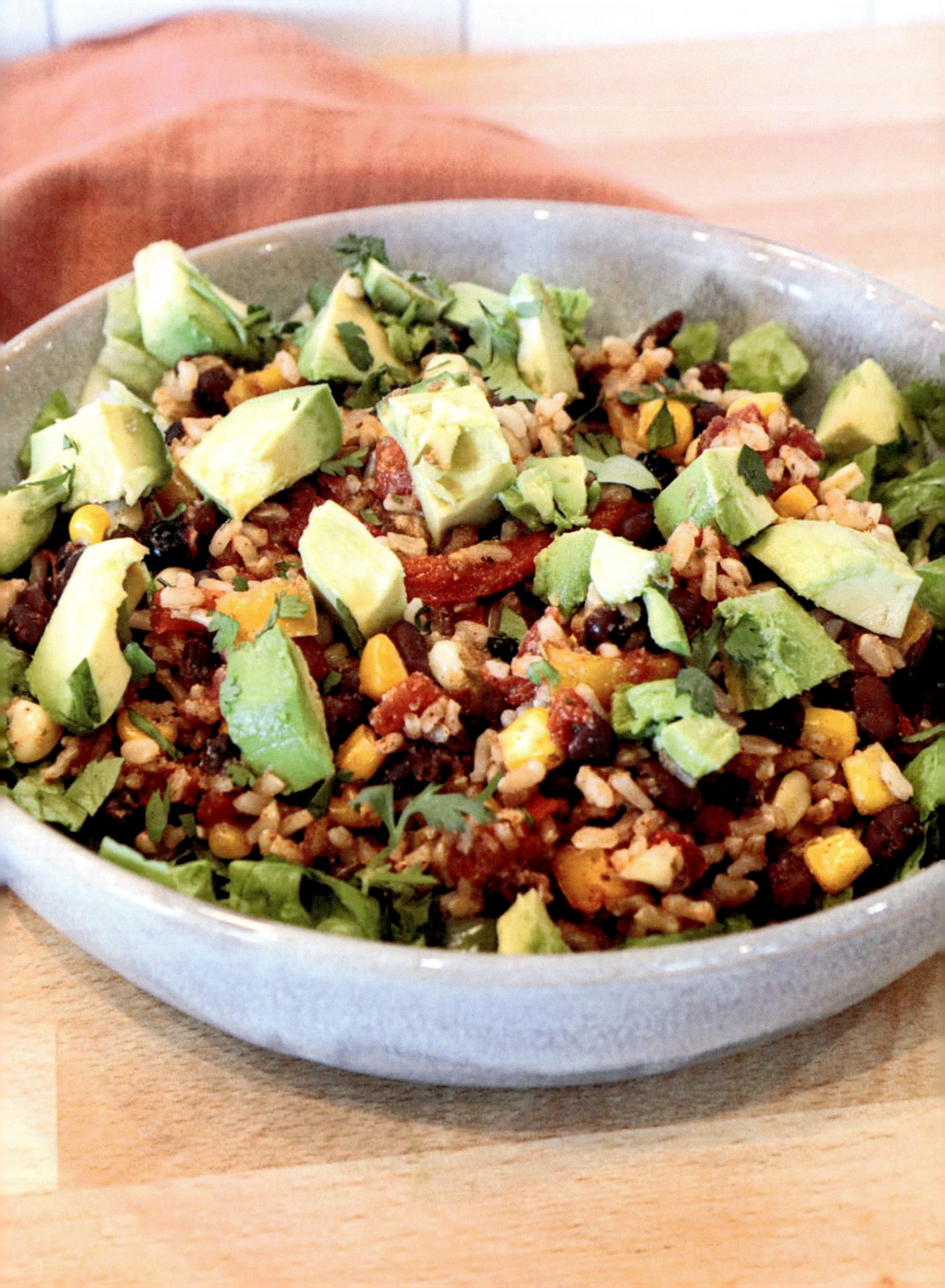

# MICROWAVED MEXICAN RICE

This travel-friendly spin on our Mexican Buddha Bowl delivers all the flavor with minimal equipment. Perfect for hotel rooms, dorm rooms, or anywhere you have access to a microwave—delicious Mexican-inspired flavors in minutes!

## INGREDIENTS

- 1 10-12 oz. bag frozen rice
- 1/2 11 oz. can fire roasted Rotel or diced tomatoes
- 1/4 15 oz. can black beans, drained and rinsed
- 1 handful frozen corn
- 1 handful frozen bell peppers
- 1 teaspoon garlic powder
- 1 teaspoon onion powder
- 1 teaspoon smoked paprika
- 1 teaspoon hatch green chili powder (optional)

### Serve With
- romaine lettuce, chopped
- salsa
- avocado

## METHOD

Add all the ingredients to a large mixing bowl and toss to combine thoroughly. Transfer to a microwave-safe bowl, cover loosely, and microwave for about 5 minutes, stirring halfway through, until everything is heated through.

Use a fork to fluff the mixture, then serve over a bed of chopped romaine. Top with fresh salsa and diced avocado for added flavor. Enjoy!

Note: For even faster prep, substitute 1-2 tablespoons of our Red or Green Chile seasoning blend for the individual spices. This recipe works great for meal prep, prepare several portions and store in microwave-safe containers for quick lunches throughout the week!

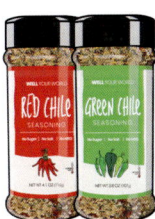

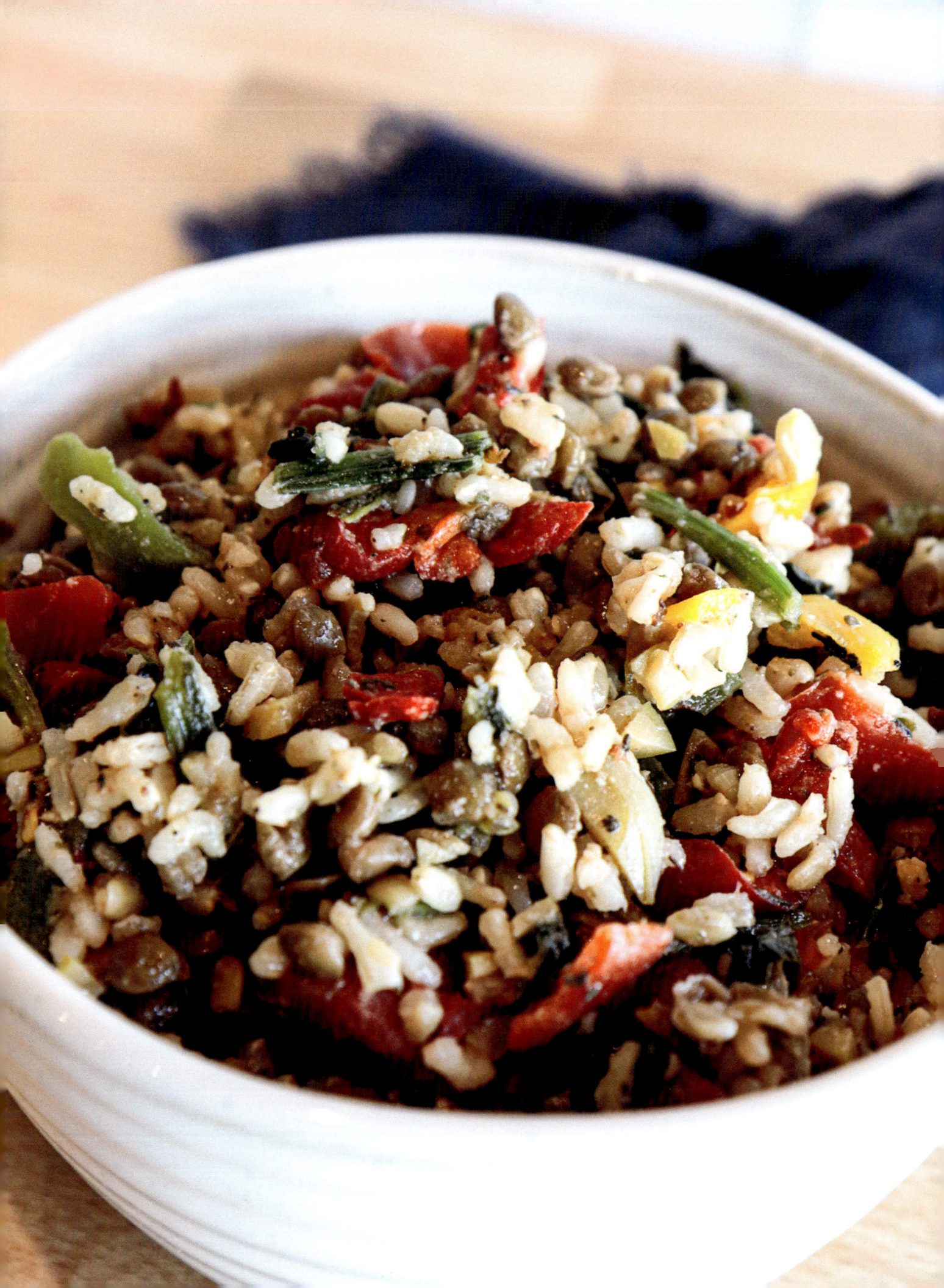

# STUFFED PEPPER BOWL

Enjoy all the classic stuffed pepper flavors without the fuss of actual stuffing! This convenient microwave meal combines protein-rich lentils, rice, and colorful vegetables with Italian herbs for a satisfying dish perfect for busy days or when you're away from home.

## INGREDIENTS

- 1/2　10-12 oz. bag frozen rice
- 1/2　15 oz. can lentils
- 1　handful frozen bell pepper strips
- 1　handful frozen chopped spinach
- 1/4　cup diced or crushed tomatoes
- 2　teaspoons nutritional yeast
- 1　teaspoon Italian seasoning
- 1　teaspoon garlic powder
- 1　teaspoon onion powder
- 1/2　teaspoon black pepper or crushed red pepper

　chopped olives, to serve (optional)

## METHOD

Add all ingredients to a large mixing bowl and toss to combine. Transfer to a microwave-safe bowl, cover with a paper towel, and microwave for about 4 minutes, stirring halfway through.

Fluff with a fork to separate the grains and distribute the flavors evenly. Top with chopped olives if desired. Enjoy!

Note: This versatile recipe works with any frozen vegetables you have on hand. The leftovers make an excellent filling for a lunch wrap the next day! And be sure to try our WYW Italian Seasoning in place of all the listed seasonings!

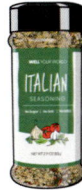

# HOW TO USE THE RECIPE CARDS

We don't like the "meal planner" method so we didn't include one in this book. Instead of telling you what to eat and when to eat it, which never works because of individual differences and moods, we want to set you up for success with FAST and EASY recipes that you can display somewhere obvious. Rely on these cards when recipe amnesia sets in!

### 1. PRINT OUT THE RECIPE CARDS ON THE NEXT PAGES

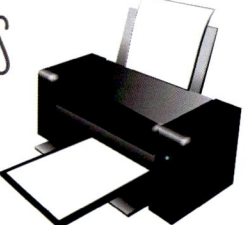

You can use the ones printed in this book or print copies from the digital e-book version. Then simply cut them out on the dotted lines! Some members of our community even laminate the cards!

### 2. HANG THE CARDS WHERE YOU CAN SEE THEM

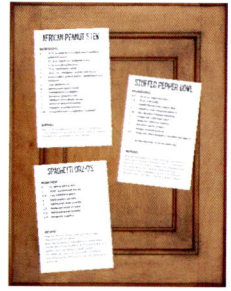

Choose 6-8 recipes to create your current meal rotation. We suggest taping them to your refrigerator, the inside of your pantry door, or anywhere in your kitchen that you see often.

### 3. FAMILIARIZE YOURSELF WITH THE INGREDIENTS

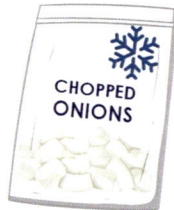

Once you start to make the same recipes over and over, you'll get a sense of what you need to have on hand in your pantry, fridge, and freezer. At our house we have one memorized list of shopping items and those ingredients work for almost every recipe we make.

### 4. MAKE SURE TO HAVE THOSE INGREDIENTS IN STOCK

Start building your family's list of everyday go-to shopping ingredients. Many of the recipes in this guide can be frozen or canned, so you don't have to worry about ingredients spoiling in the fridge.

### 5. DON'T BE AFRAID TO REPEAT MEALS!

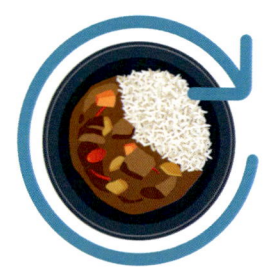

Whether it's leftovers from a big batch of something you made yesterday, or you are making your second batch of Potato Corn Chowder this week, don't be afraid to enjoy your favorite meals on repeat. This is critical to simplifying your healthy diet!

# SIMPLE CHICKPEA BRUSCHETTA

## INGREDIENTS

| | |
|---|---|
| 1 | 15 oz. can chickpeas, drained and rinsed |
| 1 | tablespoon minced garlic |
| 1/4 | teaspoon crushed red pepper (optional) |
| 2 | tablespoons tahini |
| 1 | lemon, juiced |
| 1 | handful parsley, chopped |
| 1/4 | cup sun dried tomatoes, chopped |

## METHOD

Add the chickpeas, garlic, and crushed red pepper to a mixing bowl and mash into a coarse texture with a potato masher or fork. Add the remaining ingredients and mix well. Enjoy on toast, lavash, a bed of lettuce, with carrot chips, cucumber chips, crackers, and so much more!

# CHICKPEA LETTUCE CUPS

## INGREDIENTS

| | |
|---|---|
| 1 | 15 oz. can chickpeas, drained and rinsed |
| 1 | teaspoon ground turmeric |
| 1 | teaspoon ground cumin |
| 1 | teaspoon curry powder |
| 1/2 | teaspoon chili powder |
| 1 | green onion, chopped |
| 3 | garlic cloves, minced |
| 6-8 | mint leaves, chopped |
| 1 | tablespoon sesame seeds |
| | lettuce, to serve |
| | avocado, to serve |

## METHOD

Heat up a skillet and add a few tablespoons of water along with the chickpeas, turmeric, cumin, curry, and chili powder. Stir together to coat the chickpeas.
Once the water has mostly cooked off, add the remaining ingredients and stir for about a minute. To serve, spoon the chickpea mixture onto lettuce cups and top with avocado.

# HEARTY-CHOKE SANDWICH

## INGREDIENTS

| | |
|---|---|
| 1/2 | 16 oz. bag frozen/canned artichoke hearts, thawed |
| 1 | 15 oz. can white beans, drained and rinsed |
| 3 | garlic cloves, minced |
| 1 | handful fresh basil |
| 1/2 | lemon, juiced |
| 1 | tablespoon tahini (optional) |
| 1-2 | teaspoons favorite no-salt seasoning |

### Sandwich Toppings

- whole wheat bread or lavash, toasted/warmed
- fresh spinach or lettuce
- sliced tomato
- sliced red or green onion
- black pepper

## METHOD

Add all of the ingredients to a food processor and pulse a few times. Wipe down the sides and pulse again until it reaches a slightly creamy texture. Spread the mixture on toast and add your favorite sandwich toppings. Enjoy!

# SMASHED CHICKPEA AVOCADO DIP

## INGREDIENTS

| | |
|---|---|
| 2 | 15 oz. cans chickpeas, drained and rinsed |
| 1-2 | avocados |
| 1 | jalapeño, seeded and diced |
| 3 | green onions, sliced |
| 1 | pint cherry tomatoes, halved |
| 2 | garlic cloves, minced |
| 2 | limes, juiced |
| 1/4 | cup fresh cilantro, chopped |

### Wrap Ingredients

- whole wheat lavash or tortilla
- sliced red onion
- lettuce or Cruciferous Crunch
- char-roasted corn

## METHOD

Add the chickpeas to a large mixing bowl and mash with a potato masher into a coarse, chunky texture.
Toss in the avocado and continue mashing to mix together. Add the remaining ingredients and stir to combine.
Make a wrap by adding the dip to a whole wheat lavash or tortilla and add all of the fixings you like!

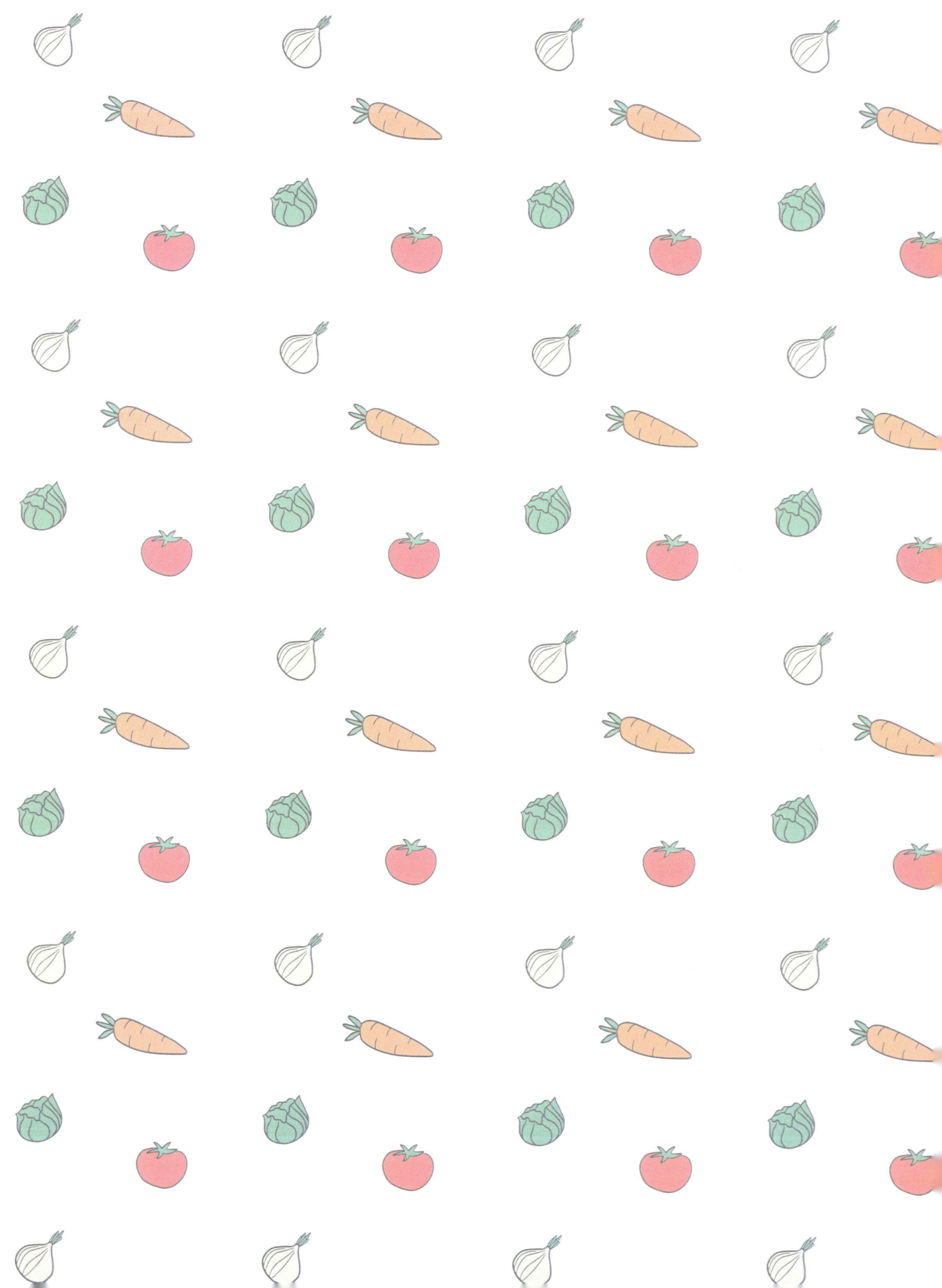

## MCREEBS WRAP

### INGREDIENTS

**McReebs Secret Sauce**
- 1/2 cup raw cashews
- 1/2 cup water
- 1/4 cup ketchup
- 1 tablespoon nutritional yeast
- 1 teaspoon dijon or yellow mustard
- 1/2 teaspoon paprika
- 1 green onion
- 1 small lemon, juiced

**Burger Mash**
- 1 15 oz. can kidney beans, drained and rinsed
- 1 tablespoon favorite spice blend

### METHOD

To prepare the McReebs Sauce, add all of the ingredients to a high-speed blender and blend until smooth.

For the Burger Mash, mash the kidney beans together with your favorite no-salt spice blend in a small bowl using a potato masher or a fork.

Lay out the lavash, spread the burger mash with other fixings of your choice (page 31), and drizzle on the McReebs Sauce. Roll it up and cut in half.

## BBQ SUMMER WRAP

### INGREDIENTS

**Chickpea Filling**
- 1 15 oz. can chickpeas, drained and rinsed
- 1/2 cup frozen fire roasted corn, thawed
- 1/2 cup BBQ sauce

**Wrap Ingredients**
- whole wheat lavash
- chickpea filling
- 1-2 ribs celery, sliced thin
- 1 red bell pepper, sliced thin
- 1 carrot, sliced thin
- 1 avocado, sliced
- 1/2 cucumber, sliced thin

### METHOD

Add the chickpeas, corn, and BBQ sauce (page 33) to a mixing bowl. Mash into a coarse texture with a potato masher.

Lay out the lavash, add some chickpea filling along with as much of the other wrap ingredients as you like, roll it up, and cut the wrap in half.

## MMMBLT WRAP

### INGREDIENTS

**Mushroom Bacon**
- 1/2 cup veggie broth
- 1/2 teaspoon liquid smoke
- 2 tablespoons balsamic vinegar
- 1 teaspoon garlic powder
- 1 teaspoon onion powder
- 1 teaspoon paprika
- 3-4 portobello mushrooms, sliced

**Dillapeño Sauce**
- 1/4 cup tahini
- 1-2 tablespoons fresh chopped dill
- 1 jalapeño, seeds removed
- 1 lime, juiced
- 1-2 deglet dates
- 2 garlic cloves
- 1+ tablespoons water, as needed
- black pepper, to taste

### METHOD

Add all of the Mushroom Bacon ingredients to a saucepan and sauté on medium-high heat until the mushrooms soften and the liquid has cooked off.

Add all of the Dillapeño Sauce ingredients to a blender, reserving about 1/2 the dill, and blend until smooth. Add the remaining dill and pulse a few times.

Lay out the lavash, add some mushrooms along with all of the other wrap ingredients (page 35). Drizzle on the Dillapeño Sauce, roll it up, and cut in half.

## SUSHIRRITO

### INGREDIENTS

- 1/2 14-16 oz. extra firm block tofu
- 1 teaspoon garlic powder
- 1 teaspoon onion powder
- 1 teaspoon sesame seeds
- 1 teaspoon soy sauce (optional)
- 1 teaspoon rice vinegar
- 1/2-1 teaspoon Sriracha
- 1 sheet nori, chopped
- 1 green onion, chopped

**Wrap Ingredients**
- cooked rice
- avocado
- carrot
- cucumber
- tofu mix
- whole wheat lavash, tortilla, or spring roll wrap

### METHOD

Crumble the tofu into a large mixing bowl using your hands. Add the remaining ingredients and toss to combine.

Lay out the wrap, add rice, and press flat. Add the other burrito ingredients, roll up, and cut in half.

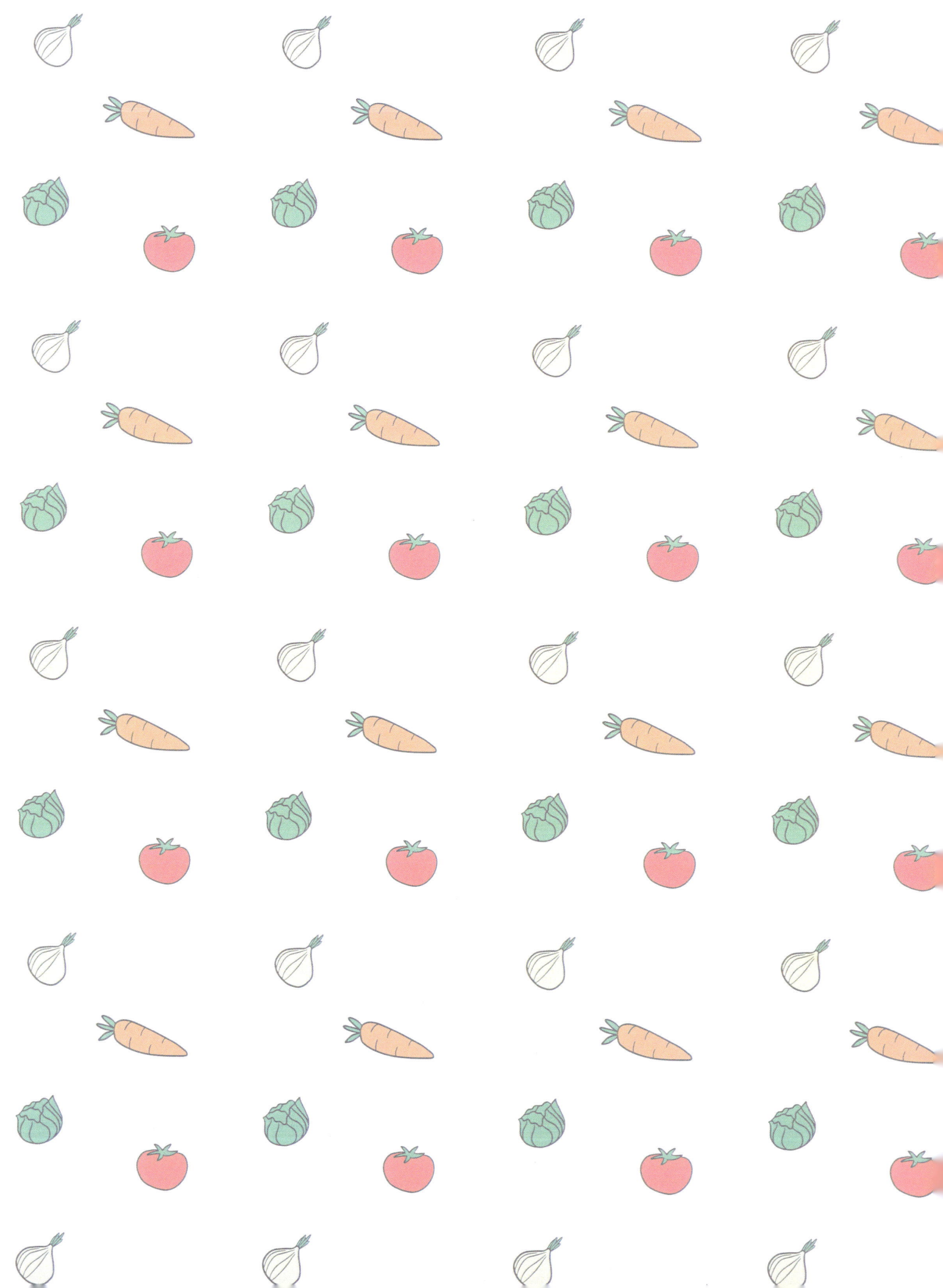

## WORLD'S FASTEST LENTIL STEW

### INGREDIENTS

| | |
|---|---|
| 12 | cups water or veggie broth |
| 3 | cups brown lentils, cooked (or 2 15 oz. cans) |
| 1/2 | cup dehydrated onion |
| 4 | tablespoons Berbere or favorite spice blend |
| 2 | 1 lb. bags frozen chopped spinach |
| 2 | 10-12 oz. bags chopped butternut squash |
| 1 | 6 oz. can tomato paste |

### METHOD

Add all of the ingredients to a large stock pot and bring to a boil. Reduce heat to medium and simmer for 5-10 minutes, stirring occasionally. (Berbere Spice Blend on page 39)

## MEXICAN FIESTA CHILI

### INGREDIENTS

| | |
|---|---|
| 2 | 15 oz. cans diced tomatoes |
| 1 | 15 oz. can tomato sauce |
| 1 | 15 oz. can pinto beans, drained and rinsed |
| 1 | 15 oz. can black beans, drained and rinsed |
| 1 | 14-16 oz. bag frozen fire roasted peppers & onions |
| 1/2 | 1 lb. bag frozen char roasted corn |
| 1 | 10-12 oz. bag frozen brown rice |
| 2 | tablespoons nutritional yeast |
| 1 | tablespoon minced garlic |
| 2 | teaspoons dried oregano |
| 1 | teaspoon dried cilantro |
| 1 | teaspoon ground cumin |
| 1 | teaspoon chipotle powder |
| 2 | teaspoons date powder |
| 1 | teaspoon crushed red pepper (optional) |

### METHOD

Add all of the ingredients to a large soup pot and heat to a boil. Reduce the heat and let simmer for 5-10 minutes.
Top with lime, fresh cilantro, and chopped olives.

## POTATO CORN CHOWDER

### INGREDIENTS

| | |
|---|---|
| 4 | cups veggie broth |
| 2 | cups soy milk |
| 1/4 | cup nutritional yeast |
| 2 | teaspoons dried parsley |
| 2 | teaspoons dried chives |
| 2 | teaspoons garlic powder |
| 1 | teaspoon dried tarragon |
| 1/2 | teaspoon black pepper |
| 1/2 | teaspoon paprika |
| 1 | 1 lb. bag frozen Potatoes O' Brien (cubed potatoes) |
| 1 | 10-12 oz. bag frozen mirepoix mix (diced carrots, celery, and onion) |
| 1 | 15 oz. can corn, drained and rinsed |

### METHOD

Add all of the ingredients to a large soup pot, heat to a boil, reduce the heat and let simmer for a few minutes.

## INDIAN CHILI

### INGREDIENTS

| | |
|---|---|
| 2 | 15 oz. cans tomato sauce |
| 1 | 15 oz. can diced tomatoes |
| 1 | 15 oz. can chickpeas, drained and rinsed |
| 1 | 1 lb. bag frozen cauliflower florets |
| 1 | 1 lb. bag frozen Potatoes O'Brien (cubed potatoes) |
| 1 | 10-12 oz. bag frozen chopped onion |
| 1 1/2 | cups frozen mixed vegetables |
| 1 | tablespoon minced garlic |
| 1 | tablespoon curry powder |
| 1 | tablespoon ground coriander |
| 1 | tablespoon date powder |
| 1 | teaspoon ground cumin |
| 1/2 | teaspoon ground turmeric |
| 1/2 | teaspoon ground chili powder |
| 1+ | cups veggie broth |

### METHOD

Add all of the ingredients to a large soup pot and bring to a boil. Reduce heat and simmer for 5-10 minutes.
Top with fresh lime and cilantro.

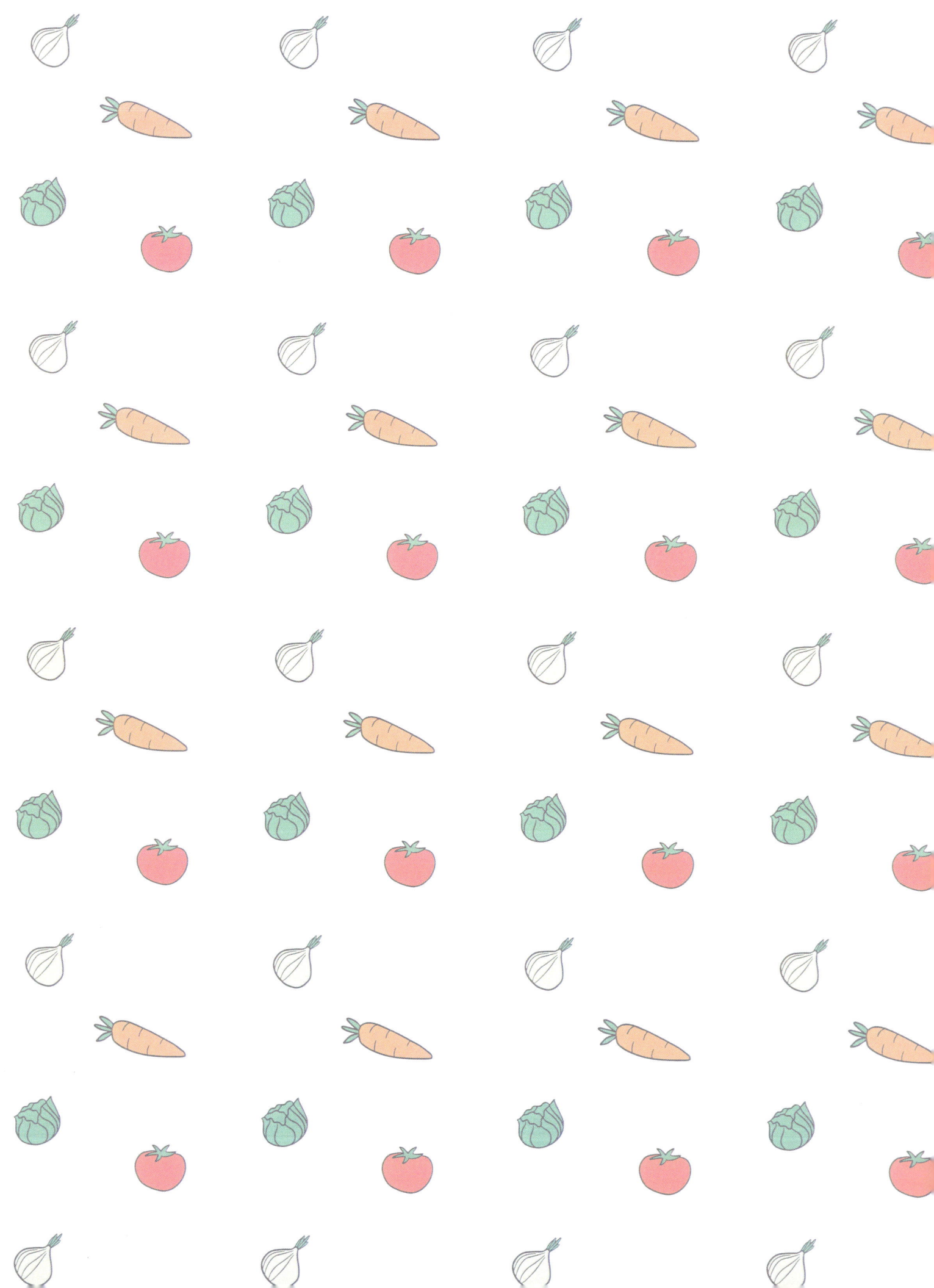

# PEANUT RAMEN BOWL

## INGREDIENTS

| | |
|---|---|
| 4-6 | tablespoons water |
| 1 | tablespoon lime juice |
| 1 | tablespoon rice vinegar |
| 1/3 | cup peanut butter |
| 1 | tablespoon soy sauce/tamari/miso (optional) |
| 2 | teaspoons date powder (or 2 deglet dates) |
| 1" | fresh ginger |
| 3 | garlic cloves |
| 1 | green onion |
| | crushed red pepper or Thai chilis, to taste |

### Serve With:
- brown rice ramen
- frozen bell pepper
- frozen edamame
- frozen broccoli
- Peanut Sauce
- sliced green onion
- chopped cilantro
- sesame seeds

## METHOD

To prepare the Peanut Sauce, add all of the ingredients to a high speed blender and blend until smooth. Set aside.

Bring a pot of water to a boil and throw in 2-3 ramen noodle blocks. Cook for about 5 minutes, using a fork to break them apart once they start to soften. Add frozen broccoli and edamame to the pot. Let it simmer a few more minutes. Drain and transfer to a bowl. Toss with the Peanut Sauce and broccoli slaw.

Top with green onions, cilantro, and sesame seeds.

# MEXICAN BUDDHA BOWL

## INGREDIENTS

| | |
|---|---|
| 1 | 10-12 oz. bag frozen brown rice |
| 1 | 14-16 oz. bag frozen "Southwest Veggies" (onions, bell peppers, corn, beans) |
| 1 | tablespoon no-salt seasoning like WYW Chili Lime or Fiesta Blend |

### Serve With:
- romaine lettuce
- pico de gallo
- chopped tomatoes
- sliced avocado
- cilantro
- lime juice

## METHOD

Add the frozen rice to a steamer basket on the stove along with the bag of frozen Southwest veggies. Sprinkle the seasoning on top of the veggies, cover, and allow to steam for 5-10 minutes to heat through.

To assemble, add a layer of chopped romaine lettuce to the bottom of a large plate or bowl and top with the steamed mix.

Top with pico de gallo, chopped tomatoes, avocado, cilantro, and lime juice.

# EGGPLANT BEAN DELIGHT

## INGREDIENTS

| | |
|---|---|
| 1 | eggplant, chopped into 1/4" cubes |
| 2 | teaspoons smoked paprika |
| 1 | teaspoon onion powder |
| 1 | teaspoon garlic powder |
| 1 | teaspoon date powder |
| 1/2 | teaspoon crushed red pepper (optional) |
| 1 | 15 oz. can white beans, drained and rinsed |
| 1 | 15 oz. can chickpeas, drained and rinsed |
| 1 | 15 oz. can diced tomatoes |
| 1 | tablespoon tomato paste |
| 1/2 | lemon, juiced |
| 1 | tablespoon tahini (optional) |
| 2 | handfuls fresh spinach |

## METHOD

Add the eggplant to a large pot and sauté over medium-high heat for 5-7 minutes until soft, adding veggie stock as needed to keep from sticking.

Add the paprika, onion powder, garlic powder, date powder, crushed red pepper, white beans, and chickpeas. Continue to sauté for a couple more minutes.

Stir in the diced tomatoes and tomato paste and heat back up to a simmer.

Add the lemon juice, tahini, and fresh spinach and mix well to cook the spinach for another minute.

# SIMPLE SEASONED LENTILS

## INGREDIENTS

| | |
|---|---|
| 2 | 15 oz. cans lentils (or 3 cups cooked) |
| 1 | 10-12 oz. bag frozen chopped onions |
| 1 | 10-12 oz. bag frozen chopped bell peppers |
| 2 | teaspoons minced garlic |
| 1-2 | tablespoons no-salt seasoning |
| 2 | tablespoons pumpkin seeds (pepitas) |
| 1 | lime, juiced |
| 1 | handful fresh greens, chopped |
| 1 | tomato, chopped |

## METHOD

Add the lentils, onion, bell peppers, and garlic to a large saucepan and sauté over medium-high heat for 5 minutes until tender, adding veggie broth as needed to keep from sticking.

Add your favorite no-salt seasoning along with the pepitas, and continue to sauté for another minute.

Squeeze on the lime and serve over a bed of greens topped with fresh chopped tomatoes.

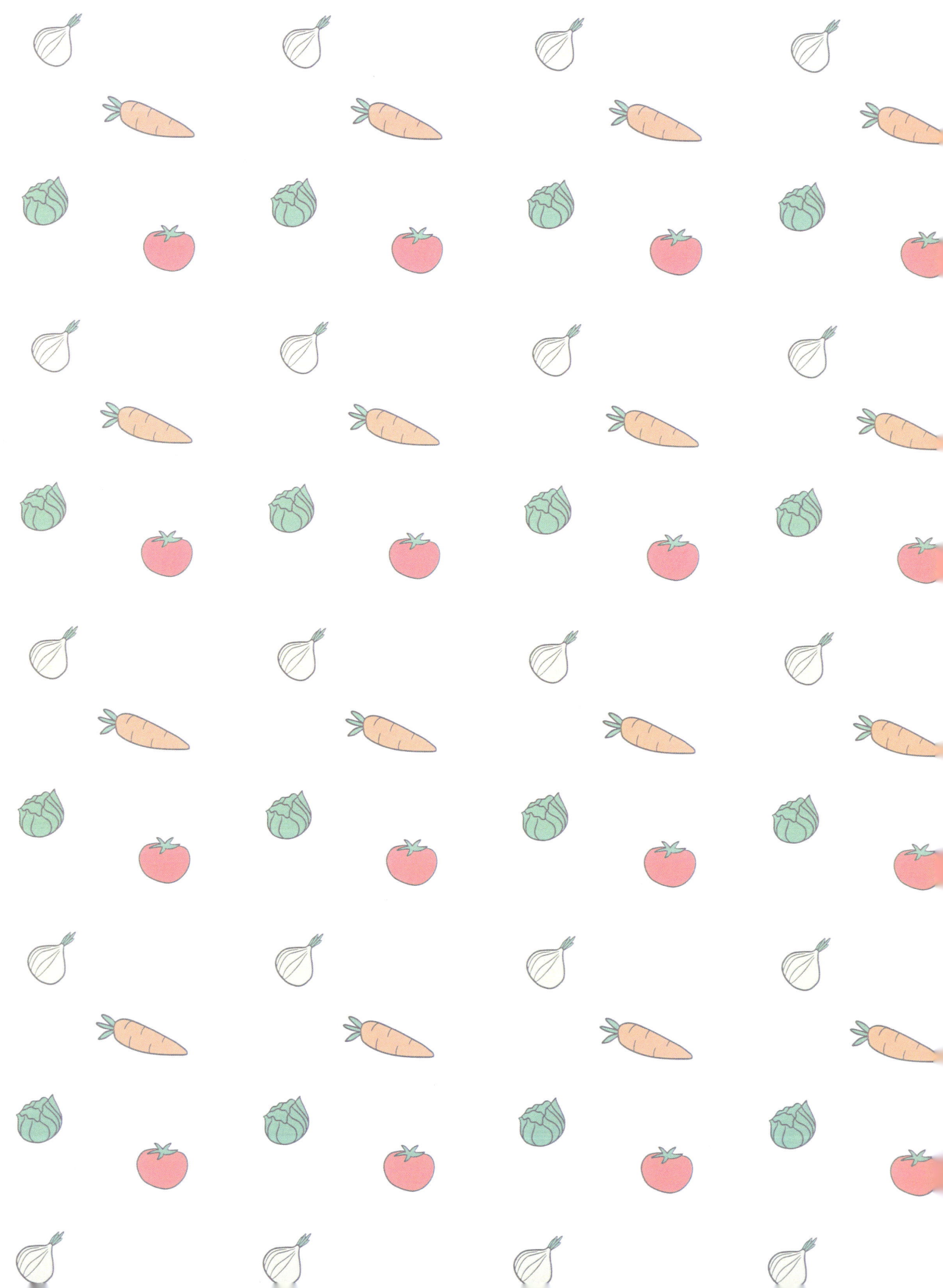

# SPEEDY BLACK EYED PEAS & GREENS

## INGREDIENTS

| | |
|---|---|
| 1 | 15 oz. can no-salt black eyed peas, drained and rinsed |
| 1 | 10-12 oz. bag frozen chopped onion |
| 2-3 | teaspoons minced garlic |
| 1-2 | tablespoons no-salt seasoning |
| 2 | big handfuls of fresh greens like kale |
| 1/2 | lemon, juiced |

## METHOD

Add the black eyed peas, onion, and garlic to a large saucepan and sauté over medium-high heat for 5-7 minutes until tender, adding veggie broth as needed to keep from sticking.
Add the no-salt seasoning and continue to sauté for another minute.
Add the greens and stir until wilted.
Squeeze fresh lemon juice over the top just before serving.

# STOVETOP WOWATOUILLE

## INGREDIENTS

| | |
|---|---|
| 1 | 10-12 oz. bag frozen brown rice |
| 1 | 10-12 oz. bag frozen peppers and onions |
| 1 | 10-12 oz. bag frozen (or 1 can) artichoke hearts |
| 2 | 15 oz. cans diced tomatoes |
| 2 | tablespoons nutritional yeast |
| 1 | tablespoon Italian seasoning |
| 2-3 | teaspoons minced garlic |
| 1 | teaspoon dried basil |
| 1 | teaspoon crushed red pepper (optional) |
| 1 | teaspoon date powder |
| 1/2 | teaspoon dried ground thyme |
| 2 | 10-12 oz. bags frozen "zoodles" (zucchini noodles) |

## METHOD

Add everything except the zoodles to a medium dutch oven over high heat. Bring to a boil while stirring occasionally, reduce the heat, and simmer for a few minutes.
Then add the zoodles since they are more fragile than the other ingredients. Stir to bring it all together, simmer to cook through for a minute or two.

# CURRIED POTATO STEW

## INGREDIENTS

| | |
|---|---|
| 2 | 15 oz. cans diced tomatoes |
| 2 | 15 oz. cans chickpeas, rinsed and drained |
| 1 | 10-12 oz. bag frozen cauliflower florets |
| 1/2 | 16 oz. bag frozen peas |
| 1/2 | 10-12 oz. bag frozen yellow onion |
| 2-3 | tablespoons curry powder |
| 1 | tablespoon minced garlic |
| 1 | tablespoon nutritional yeast |
| 1 | teaspoon chili powder |
| 1/2 | 1 lb. bag frozen cubed potatoes |

fresh chopped cilantro, to serve

## METHOD

Add everything except the potatoes to a large pot and bring to a boil. Reduce the heat and simmer for a minute, then toss in the potatoes and let simmer for a couple more minutes, stirring occasionally until potatoes are just tender.

Top with fresh chopped cilantro and enjoy!

# PASTA CARBONARA

## INGREDIENTS

| | |
|---|---|
| 1/2 | lb. whole wheat spaghetti |
| 1 | 10-12 oz. bag frozen chopped zucchini |

**Sauce**

| | |
|---|---|
| 1/2 | lb. fresh or frozen chopped mushrooms |
| 1/2 | teaspoon liquid smoke |
| 2 | cups soy milk |
| 1/4 | cup nutritional yeast |
| 1/4 | cup sun-dried tomatoes, chopped |
| 1 | tablespoon chickpea flour |
| 1 | tablespoon capers or lemon juice |
| 2-3 | teaspoons minced garlic |
| 2 | teaspoons onion powder |
| 1/4 | teaspoon black pepper |
| 1/4 | teaspoon ground nutmeg |
| 1/4 | teaspoon dried thyme |
| 1/2 | cup fresh chopped parsley |
| 2 | tablespoons pine nuts (optional) |

## METHOD

Cook the pasta according to package directions. During the last two minutes, add frozen zucchini. Drain and set aside.
Add the mushrooms to a saucepan and sauté with veggie broth for a couple minutes. Add the liquid smoke and sauté until mushrooms shrink. Whisk in soy milk and remaining ingredients except the parsley and pine nuts.
Bring sauce to a boil, reduce heat, and simmer for a few minutes. Mix in the parsley.
Toss pasta and zucchini with the sauce, stir to combine, and top with pine nuts.

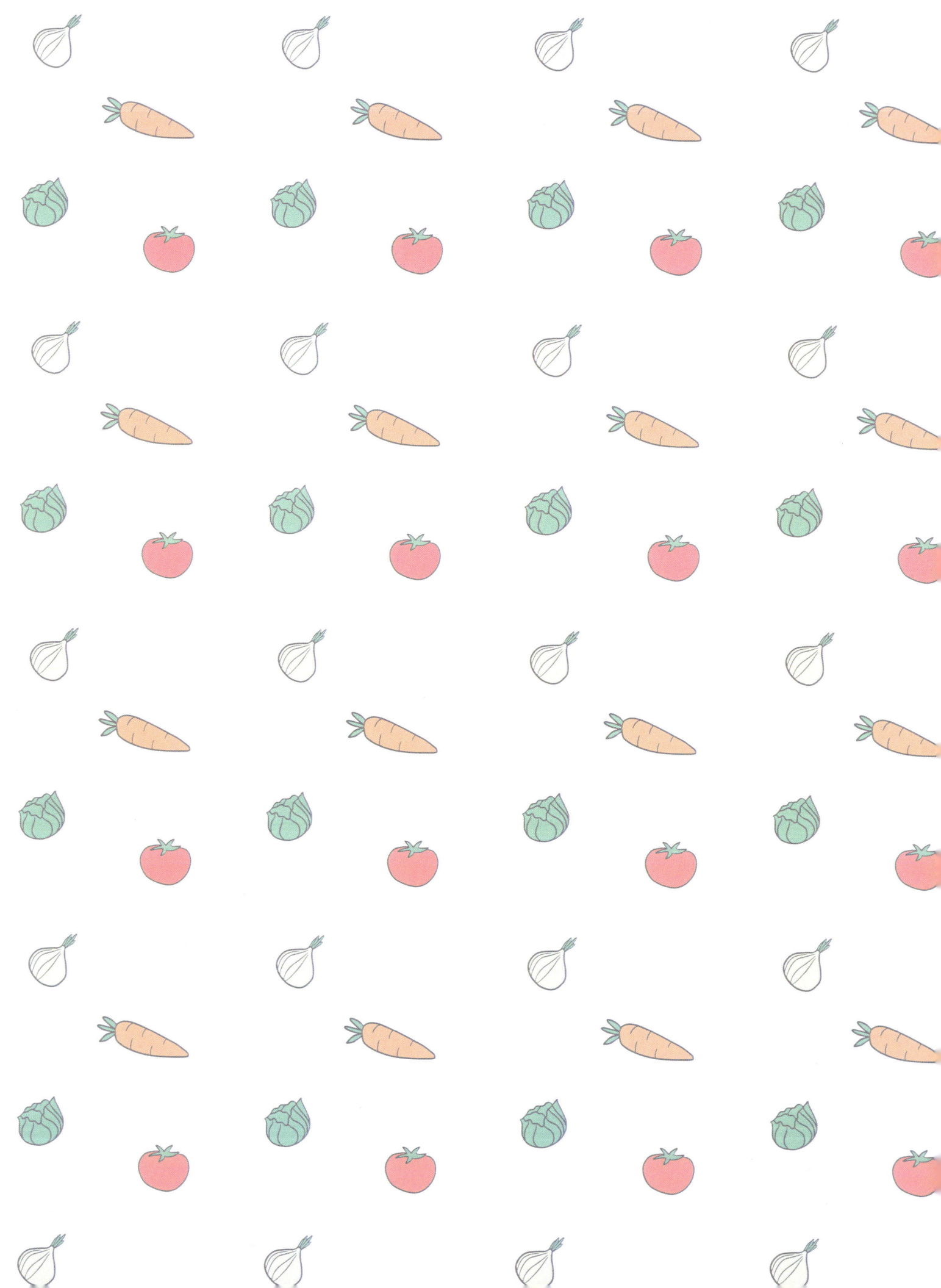

# TERIYAKI STIR FRY

## INGREDIENTS

**Teriyaki Sauce**
| | |
|---|---|
| 1/4 | cup frozen pineapple, thawed |
| 5 | tablespoons water |
| 3 | tablespoons rice vinegar |
| 1 | tablespoon tamari (optional) |
| 1 | teaspoon sriracha |
| 6 | deglet dates |
| 2 | garlic cloves |
| 1 | green onion |
| 1/2" | nub fresh ginger |

**Stir Fry**
| | |
|---|---|
| 1-2 | blocks ramen noodles |
| 1 | large handful fresh snow peas |
| 1/2 | 14-16 oz. bag frozen onion and bell pepper mix |
| 1/2 | 14-16 oz. bag frozen San Fran Blend (green beans, broccoli, onions, mushrooms, and red bell pepper) |
| 1/4 | 14-16 oz. bag frozen peas and carrots mix |
| 1/2 | 8 oz. can water chestnuts, drained |

## METHOD

Add all of the Teriyaki Sauce ingredients to a small bullet blender and blend until smooth.

Bring a pot of water to a boil and add ramen noodles. Cook according to package directions. During final 2-3 minutes, add all the frozen and canned vegetables and cook until noodles are tender and vegetables heated through.

Drain the veggies and noodles, add back to the pot with the Teriyaki Sauce. Cook for another minute or two. Top with green onions and sesame seeds.

# VEGGIE FAJITAS

## INGREDIENTS

**Veggie Fajitas**
| | |
|---|---|
| 1 | 10-12 oz. bag frozen bell pepper and onion strips |
| 1 | portobello mushroom, sliced |
| 1 | 15 oz. can black beans, drained and rinsed |
| 1/2 | cup frozen char roasted corn |
| 1 | teaspoon ground cumin |
| 2 | teaspoons dried oregano |
| 1 | teaspoon paprika |
| 1/2 | teaspoon chili powder |

**I-Need-A Fajita Sauce**
| | |
|---|---|
| 1/4 | cup tahini |
| 2 | teaspoons nutritional yeast |
| 1 | teaspoon garlic powder |
| 1 | teaspoon onion powder |
| 1/2 | teaspoon paprika |
| 1/2 | teaspoon cayenne pepper |
| 2 | deglet dates |
| 1/2 | lime, juiced |
| | water to reach desired consistency |

## METHOD

Add all of the Veggie Fajita ingredients to a large skillet and sauté with veggie broth until vegetables are tender, about 5-7 minutes.

Add all of the sauce ingredients to a blender and blend until smooth, adding water to reach desired consistency.

Stack fajita veggies on corn tortilla with sauce, pico, slaw, avocado, and cilantro.

# REEBS' RICED CAULIFLOWER

## INGREDIENTS

| | |
|---|---|
| 1 | 10-12 oz. bag frozen riced cauliflower |
| 3/4 | cup soy milk |
| 1/4 | cup nutritional yeast |
| 2 | teaspoons dried oregano |
| 1 | teaspoon onion powder |
| 1/2-1 | teaspoon chili powder |
| 1/2 | teaspoon ground cumin |

## METHOD

Add all of the ingredients to a small saucepan, stir well to combine, and simmer over medium heat for 4-6 minutes or until heated through.

For a more filling meal, sub the cauliflower for a bag of frozen rice or use a combination of both.

# CREAMY BUTTER BEANS

## INGREDIENTS

| | |
|---|---|
| 1 | 10-12 oz. bag frozen chopped onion |
| 6-8 | mushrooms, chopped (optional) |
| 1/2 | pint cherry tomatoes |
| 3 | garlic cloves, minced |
| 2 | teaspoons date powder |
| 1/2 | teaspoon liquid smoke (optional) |
| 1/4 | teaspoon crushed red pepper (optional) |
| 1/4 | teaspoon black pepper |
| 3 | tablespoons Hummus (page 69) |
| 2 | handfuls baby spinach |
| 1 | 15 oz. can butter beans, drained and rinsed |
| 1 | lemon, juiced to serve |

## METHOD

Add the onion, mushrooms, and tomatoes to a pan and sauté with veggie broth for a few minutes.

Add the garlic, date powder, liquid smoke, crushed red pepper, and black pepper, and sauté for a couple minutes. Stir in the Hummus and sauté for another minute.

Add the spinach and butter beans. Once the spinach wilts, remove from heat. Stir in lemon juice.

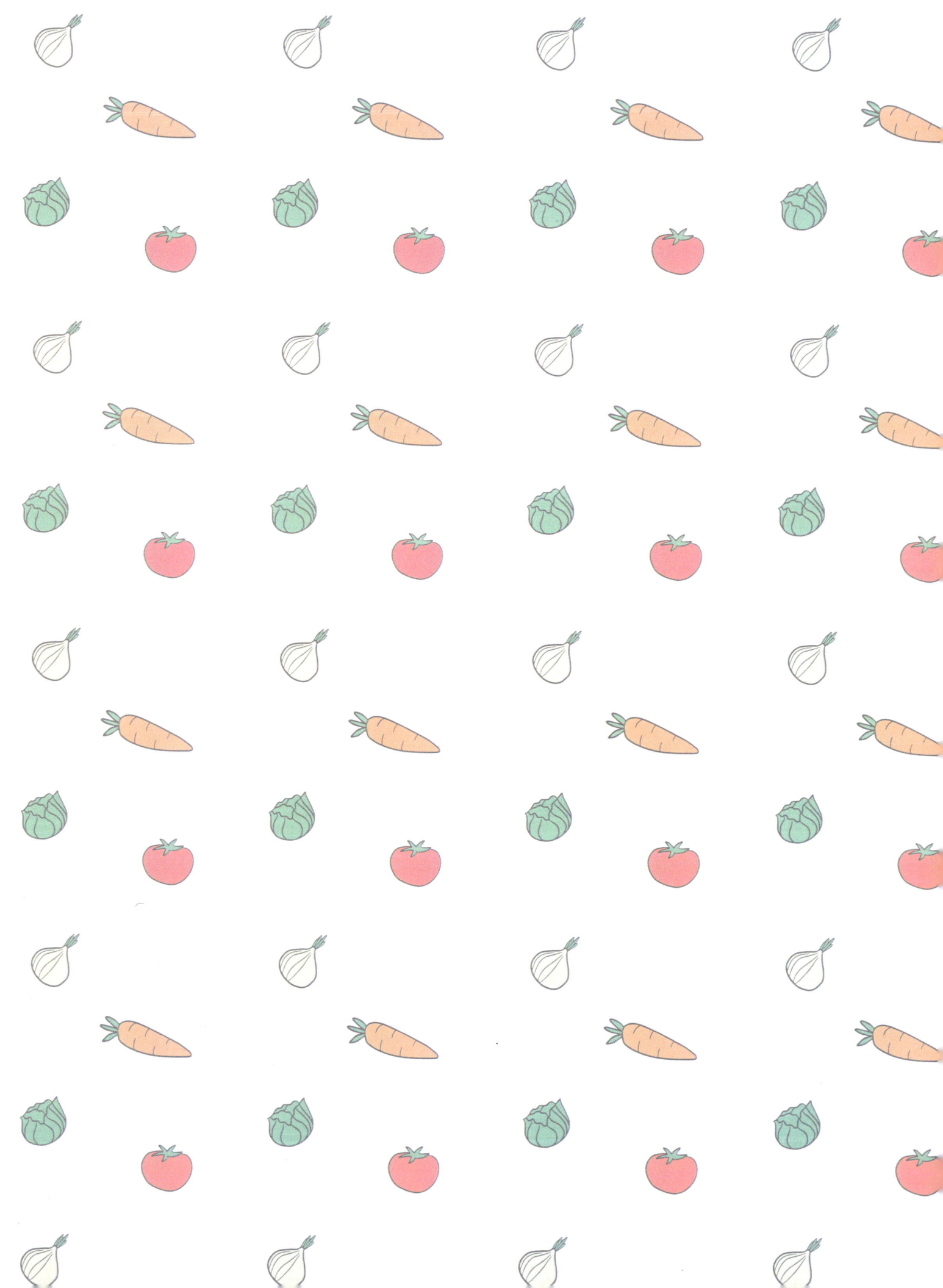

# SPAGHETTI ORZ-O'S

## INGREDIENTS
| | |
|---|---|
| 5 | oz. whole wheat orzo |
| 1 | 15 oz. can tomato sauce |
| 1/4 | cup nutritional yeast |
| 2 | tablespoons soy milk |
| 1 | tablespoon date powder |
| 1/2 | teaspoon onion powder |
| 1/2 | teaspoon garlic powder |
| 1/2 | teaspoon paprika |

## METHOD
Prepare the pasta according to package directions and set aside.
Add the remaining ingredients to a separate saucepan. Whisk together and slowly bring to a gentle boil over medium heat, stirring occasionally. Use a lid to prevent splattering.
Add the pasta to the sauce, stir, and simmer for a minute.

# MICROWAVE FRIED RICE

## INGREDIENTS
| | |
|---|---|
| 1 | 10-12 oz. bag frozen rice |
| 1 | handful frozen peas |
| 1 | handful frozen chopped kale |
| 1 | handful shredded carrots |
| 1 | handful coleslaw mix (cabbage) |
| 1 | tablespoon rice vinegar |
| 1 | tablespoon peanut butter (optional) |
| 1-2 | teaspoons tamari (optional) |
| 1 | teaspoon garlic powder |
| 1 | teaspoon onion powder |
| 1 | teaspoon ground ginger |
| 1 | teaspoon ground cumin |
| 1/4 | teaspoon ground turmeric |

chopped green onion, to serve
sesame seeds, to serve

## METHOD
Add all ingredients to a large mixing bowl and toss until well combined. Transfer to a microwave-safe bowl and microwave uncovered for about 5 minutes, stopping halfway to stir.
Fluff rice with a fork then top with chopped green onions and sesame seeds.

# SWEET POTATO BLACK BEAN BOWL

## INGREDIENTS
| | |
|---|---|
| 1 | large sweet potato, cooked, peeled, cubed, and cooled |
| 1 | 15 oz. can black beans, drained and rinsed |
| 2 | cups frozen mango, thawed and chopped |
| 1 | red bell pepper, diced |
| 1 | avocado, diced |
| 1 | handful cilantro, chopped |
| 1 | jalapeño, seeded and diced (optional) |
| 1 | lime, juiced |
| 1-2 | teaspoons WYW Chili Lime Seasoning (optional) |
| 1-2 | teaspoons WYW Calypso Seasoning (optional) |

balsamic vinegar, to taste

## METHOD
If you don't have pre-cooked sweet potatoes, boil cubed sweet potato for about 10 minutes or until tender. Drain and let cool before using.
Add all the ingredients except the balsamic vinegar to a bowl and toss gently to combine. Drizzle with balsamic vinegar and toss to coat.

# STUFFED SWEET POTATOES

## INGREDIENTS
**Chipotle Aioli**
| | |
|---|---|
| 1/2 | cup cashews |
| 1/2 | cup soy milk + tablespoon as needed |
| 1 1/2 | teaspoons chipotle powder |
| 2 | garlic cloves |
| 2 | deglet dates |
| 1 | lime, juiced |

**Stuffed Sweet Potatoes**
| | |
|---|---|
| 4 | sweet potatoes |
| 1 | 15 oz. can pinto beans, drained and rinsed |
| 1 | 12-14 oz. bag frozen char roasted onion & bell peppers |
| 1/2 | cup frozen char roasted corn |
| 1 | teaspoon ground cumin |
| 1 | teaspoon smoked paprika |
| 1 | teaspoon dried oregano |
| 1/2 | teaspoon crushed red pepper or black pepper, to taste |

## METHOD
Add all of the Chipotle Aioli ingredients to a high-speed blender and blend until smooth.
Poke holes in the sweet potatoes with a fork. Microwave two at a time for 5-7 minutes, turning halfway through, until they yield when squeezed.
Add the remaining ingredients to a saucepan. Sauté with veggie broth until heated through, about 5 minutes.
Make lengthwise cut in sweet potatoes and spoon in filling.
Top with cherry tomatoes, cilantro, coleslaw mix, and Chipotle Aioli.

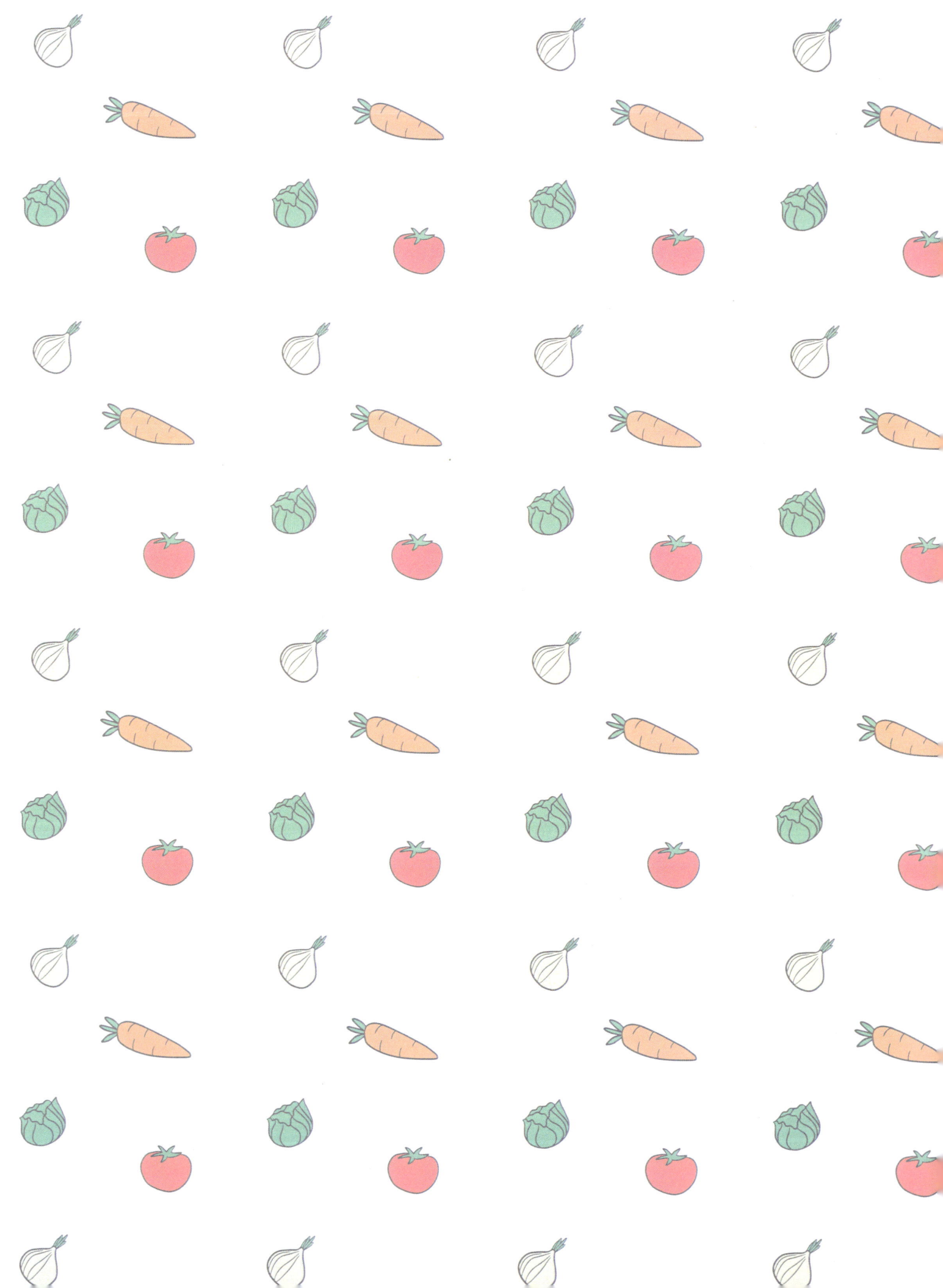

# AFRICAN PEANUT STEW

## INGREDIENTS

- 2    10-12 oz. bags frozen cubed sweet potato or butternut squash
- 1    10-12 oz. bag frozen chopped onion
- 1    15 oz. can diced tomatoes
- 1    15 oz. can tomato sauce
- 1    15 oz. can chickpeas, drained and rinsed
- 1    bunch collard greens or kale, destemmed and chopped
- 4    cups veggie broth
- 2    tablespoons peanut butter
- 1    tablespoon minced garlic
- 2    teaspoons ground cumin
- 1    teaspoon dried ground ginger
- 1    teaspoon ground cinnamon
- 1    teaspoon ground coriander
- 1/4    teaspoon crushed red pepper (optional)

## METHOD

Add all of the ingredients to a large pot and bring to a boil, stirring occasionally to prevent sticking. Reduce the heat and let simmer for 5-30 minutes.

# MUSHROOM STROGANOFF

## INGREDIENTS

- 8    oz. whole wheat or bean pasta
- 1    10-12 oz. bag frozen chopped onion
- 1    16 oz. package fresh sliced mushrooms
- 1    tablespoon minced garlic
- 2    tablespoons nutritional yeast
- 1    tablespoon white wine vinegar or lemon juice
- 1    tablespoon dijon mustard
- 1-2    teaspoons tamari (optional)
- 1/2    teaspoon dried thyme
- 1/2    teaspoon black pepper
- 1/2    teaspoon smoked paprika
- 1    cup soy milk
- 1    cup veggie broth
- 2    tablespoons whole wheat flour
- 1    handful fresh parsley, chopped

## METHOD

Prepare pasta according to package directions and set aside.
Add the onions, mushrooms, and garlic to a saucepan and sauté with veggie broth for 3-5 minutes until mushrooms release moisture and brown.
Add nutritional yeast through paprika and continue to sauté for a couple more minutes.
Add the soy milk and veggie broth, and stir well. Gradually sprinkle and whisk in the flour to prevent lumps. Simmer for 2-3 minutes until sauce thickens.
Add the pasta to saucepan and stir to combine. Serve topped with parsley and more black pepper.

# MICROWAVE MEXICAN RICE

## INGREDIENTS

- 1    10-12 oz. bag frozen rice
- 1/2    11 oz. can fire roasted Rotel or diced tomatoes
- 1/4    15 oz. can black beans, drained and rinsed
- 1    handful frozen corn
- 1    handful frozen bell peppers
- 1    teaspoon garlic powder
- 1    teaspoon onion powder
- 1    teaspoon smoked paprika
- 1    teaspoon hatch green chili powder (optional)

     chopped romaine lettuce, to serve
     salsa, to serve
     avocado, to serve

## METHOD

Add all the ingredients to a large mixing bowl and toss to combine thoroughly. Transfer to a microwave-safe bowl, cover loosely, and microwave for about 5 minutes, stirring halfway through.
Use a fork to fluff the mixture, then serve over a bed of chopped romaine. Top with fresh salsa and diced avocado for a complete meal.

# STUFFED PEPPER BOWL

## INGREDIENTS

- 1/2    10-12 oz. bag frozen rice
- 1/2    15 oz. can lentils
- 1    handful frozen bell pepper strips
- 1    handful frozen chopped spinach
- 1/4    cup diced or crushed tomatoes
- 2    teaspoons nutritional yeast
- 1    teaspoon Italian seasoning
- 1    teaspoon garlic powder
- 1    teaspoon onion powder
- 1/2    teaspoon black pepper or crushed red pepper

     chopped olives, to serve (optional)

## METHOD

Add all ingredients to a large mixing bowl and toss to combine. Transfer to a microwave-safe bowl, cover with a paper towel, and microwave for about 4 minutes, stirring halfway through.
Fluff with a fork to separate grains and distribute flavors evenly. Top with chopped olives if desired.

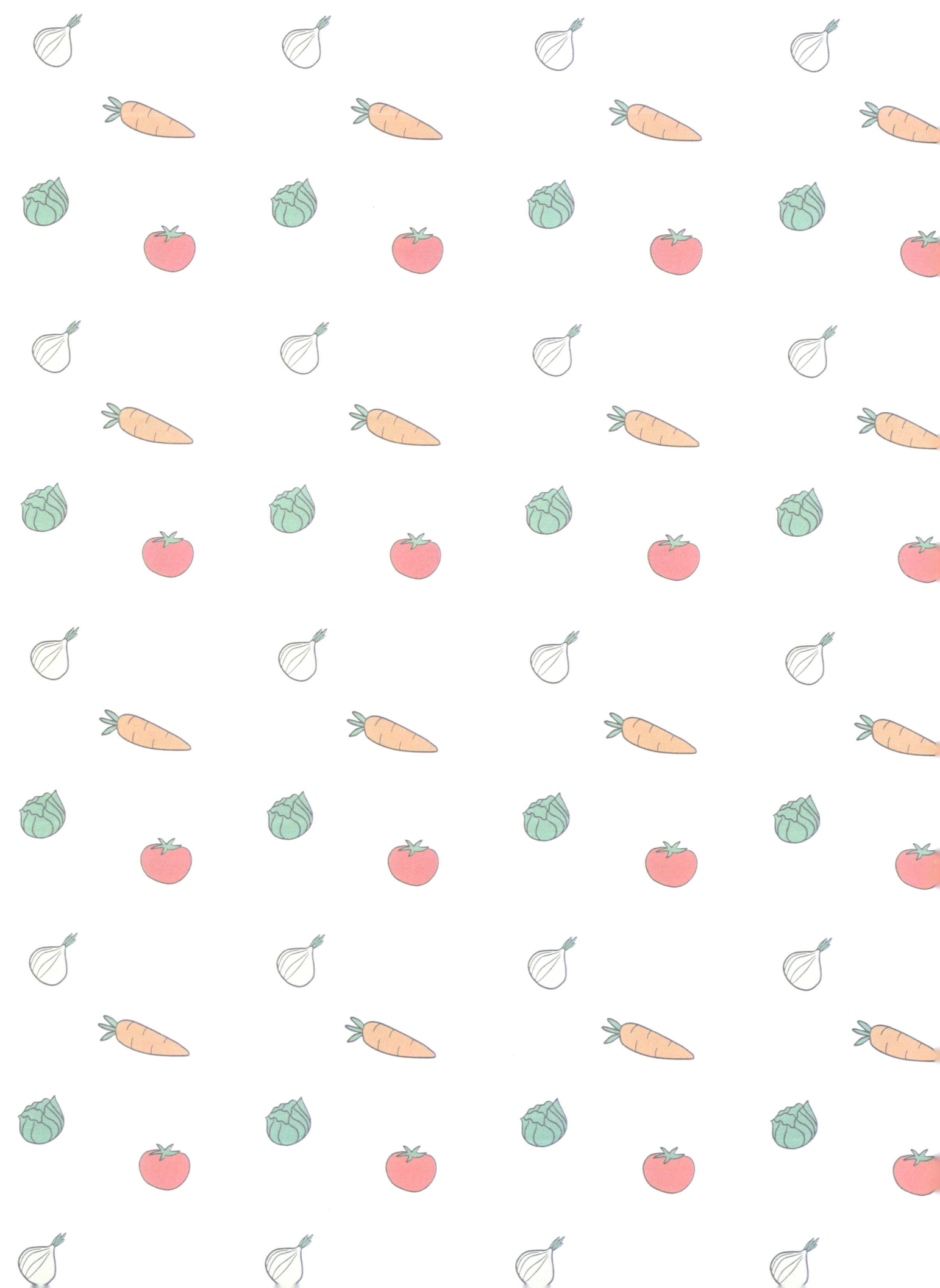

# THANK YOU!

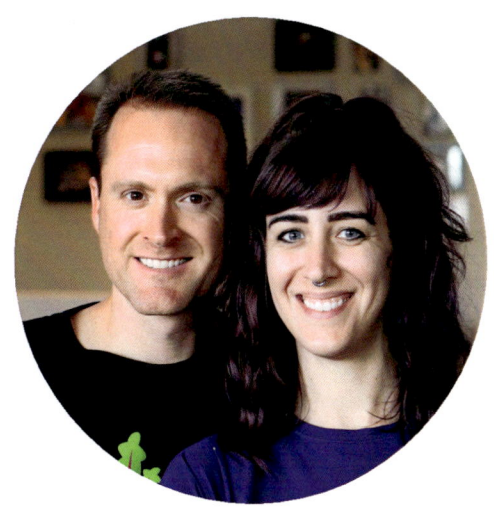

## A sincere thank you for your support!

Thank you so much for ALL you do to support us, whether it's purchasing this book, watching our YouTube videos, liking an Instagram post, or ordering our products.

We are so grateful to have a like-minded community of awesome people who appreciate all of the hard work we put into eating healthy and having fun!

If you have any questions or comments, you can always email us at: hello@wellyourworld.com

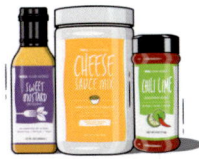

▶ youtube.com/@wellyourworld
f facebook.com/groups/wellyourworld
◉ @wellyourworld
✉ hello@wellyourworld.com

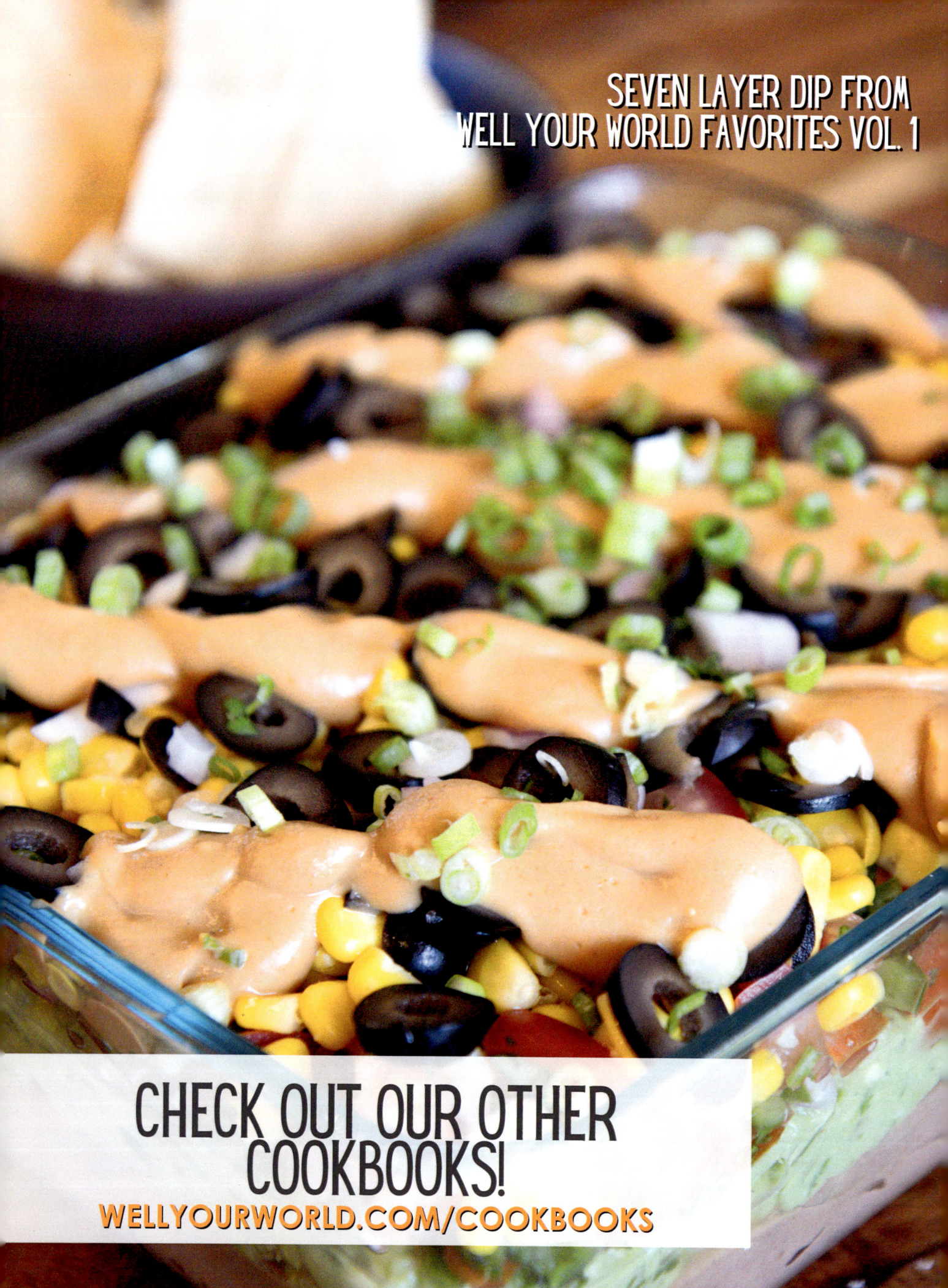

# PURCHASE OUR OTHER COOKBOOKS!

Looking for more inspiration in the kitchen? Check out our other five cookbooks, all with full color photos for each recipe, available in digital or hardcopy format. Packed with simple, no-fuss ingredients and methods, our cookbooks will help you simplify your healthy diet!

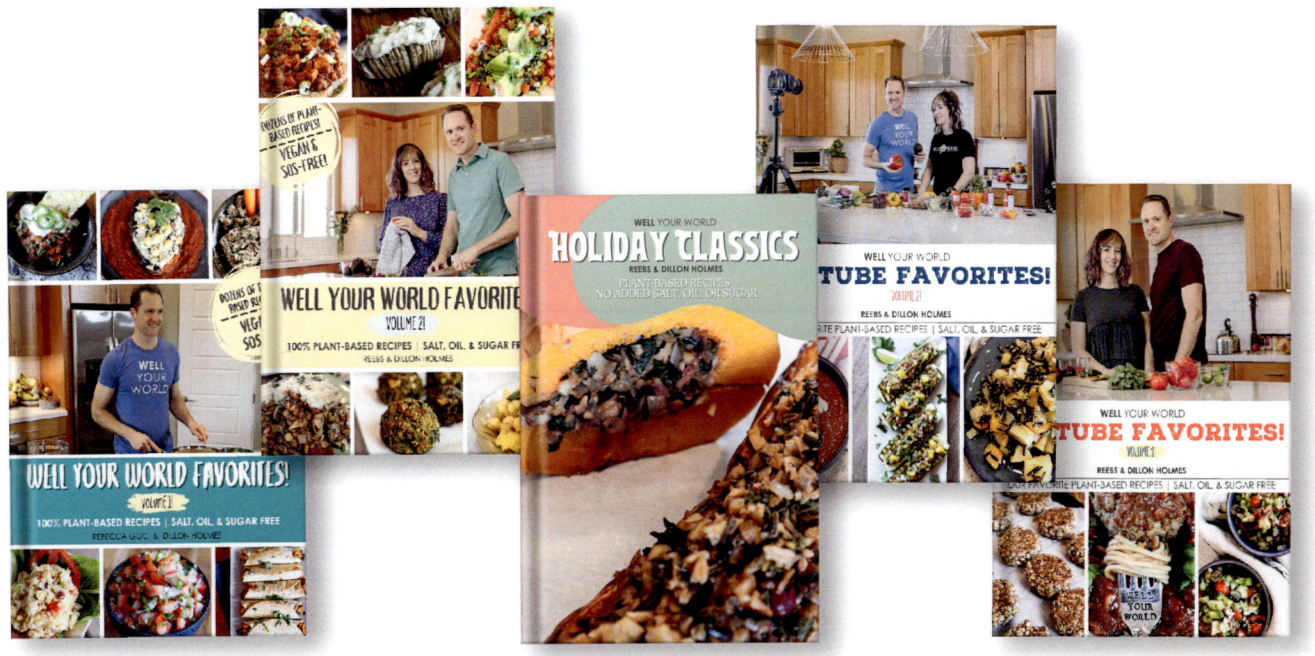

## ALL OF OUR COOKBOOKS HAVE:

- BEAUTIFUL FULL PAGE PHOTOS FOR EVERY RECIPE
- EASY TO FIND INGREDIENTS
- DOZENS OF WHOLE FOOD PLANT-BASED AND SALT, OIL, AND SUGAR FREE RECIPES
- EASY TO FOLLOW INSTRUCTIONS FOR BEGINNERS AND VETERANS ALIKE
- PAPERBACK AND DIGITAL FORMATS AVAILABLE
- TIPS AND TRICKS FOR A PLANT-BASED LIFESTYLE
- FREE SHIPPING TO THE USA

**SHOP NOW!**

↳ WELLYOURWORLD.COM/COOKBOOKS

# JOIN OUR LIVE COOKING SHOW!

If you love delicious, plant-based, SOS-free recipes like the ones in this cookbook, you'll LOVE our live interactive cooking show. We go live twice a month and create 3-4 new recipes every show. Members get access to all past replays and recipe PDF's as well as a 10% discount on ALL store products, even sale items.

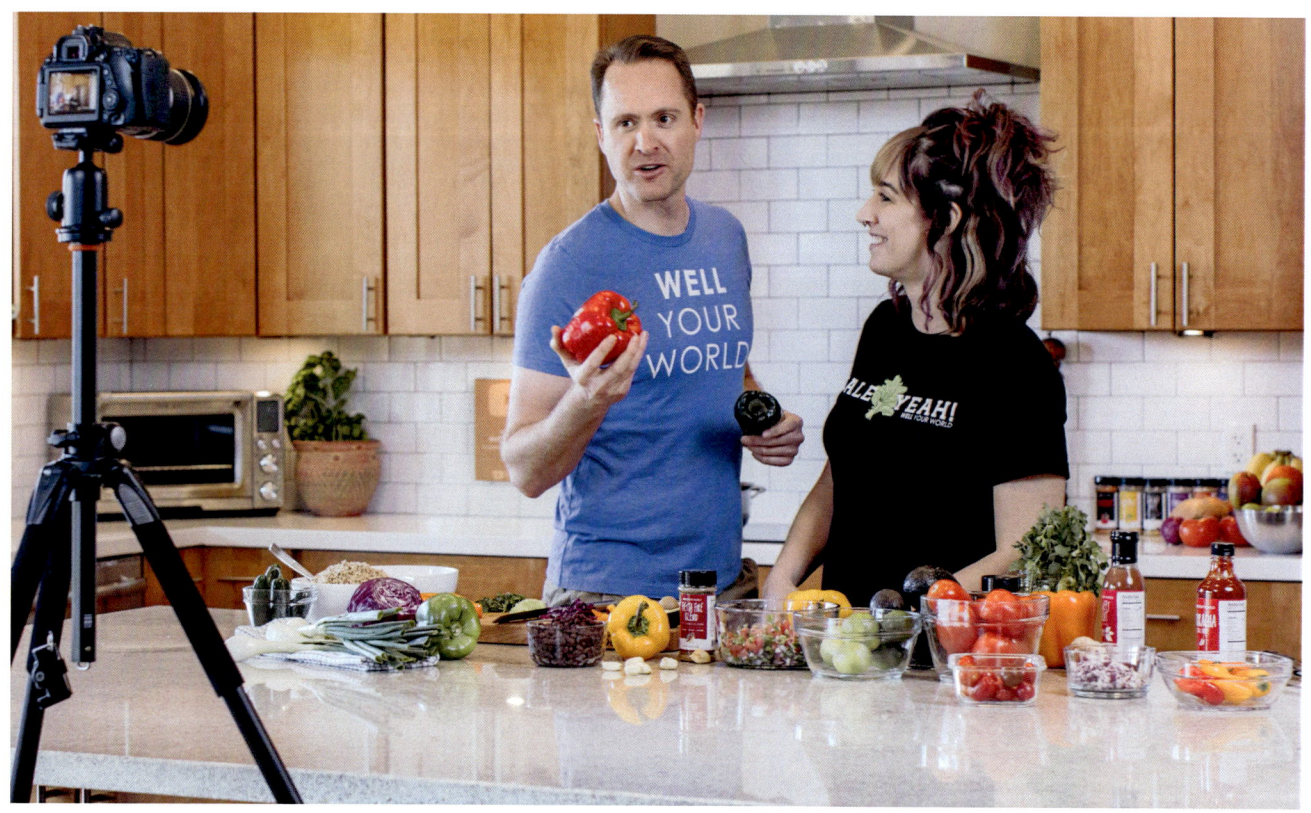

## BENEFITS OF BEING A MEMBER:

- 2 ENTERTAINING LIVE COOKING SHOWS EVERY MONTH
- 10% MEMBERS-ONLY DISCOUNT ON ALL PRODUCTS
- ACCESS TO HUNDREDS OF HEALTHY, OIL-FREE RECIPES
- OVER 175+ PAST EPISODE REPLAY VIDEOS
- RECIPE PDF DOWNLOADS FOR ALL EPISODES
- HAVE FUN WITH OTHERS WHO EAT JUST LIKE YOU!
- $15/MONTH, CANCEL ANYTIME!

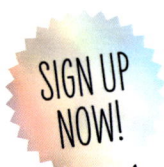
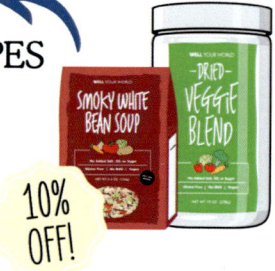

**WELLYOURWORLD.COM/COOKINGSHOW**

# SIMPLIFY YOUR DIET WITH WELL YOUR WORLD PRODUCTS!

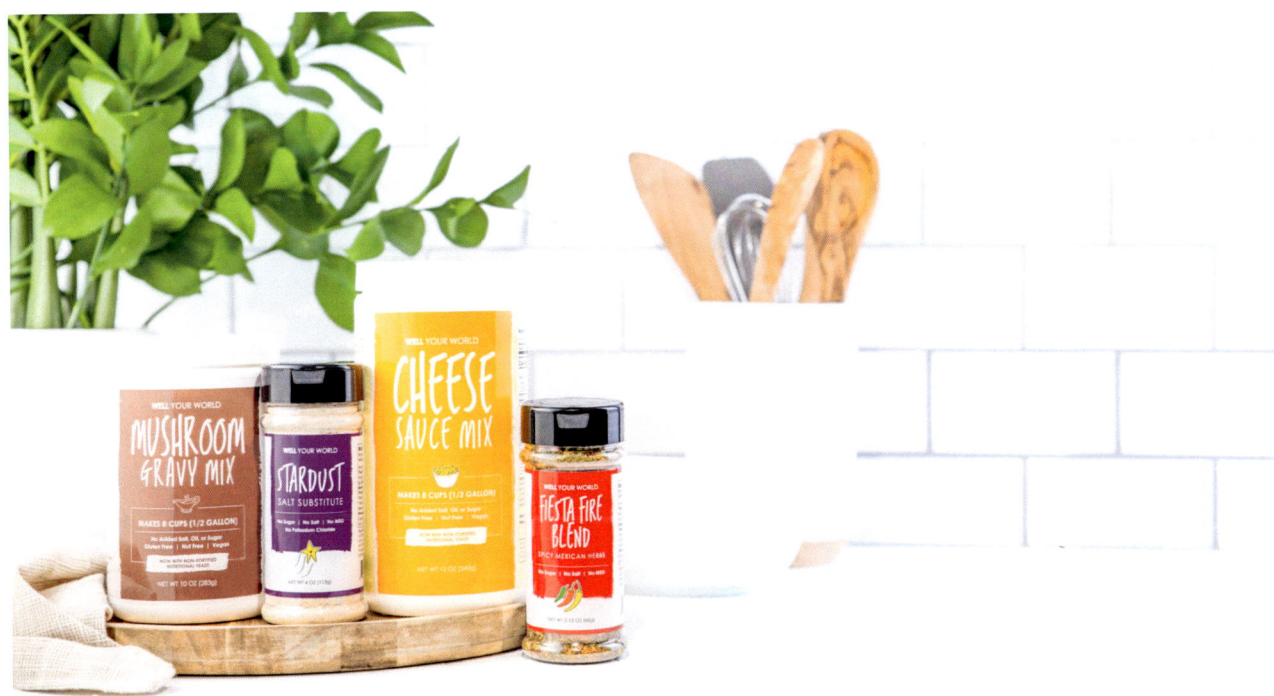

Now you can simplify your healthy diet without sacrificing time or flavor with our Well Your World lineup of whole food products.

Our time-saving pantry items make it easy to stay on track thanks to staples like our Cheese Sauce Mix, spice blends, and simmer sauces.

Check out our complete line of sauces, spices, mixes, dressings and more!

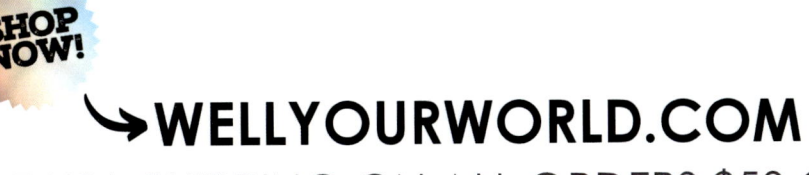

↳WELLYOURWORLD.COM

FREE USA SHIPPING ON ALL ORDERS $50 OR MORE!